MW00899871

SUPREME

MEDITERRANEAN DIET

Cookbook 2024

Super Easy, Nutritious Mediterranean Recipes to Enjoy Every Meal
and Lifelong Health with 4-Week Meal Plan for Beginners

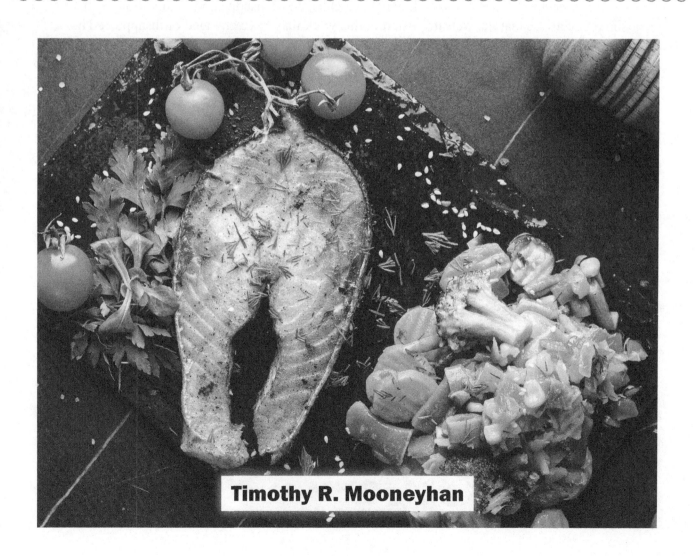

Timothy R. Mooneyhan

Copyright © 2024 Author Timothy R. Mooneyhan

Limitation of Liability/Disclaimer:

The publisher and author make no representations or warranties as to the accuracy or completeness of the contents of this work and expressly disclaim all warranties, including but not limited to warranties of fitness for a particular purpose. No warranty shall be made or enlarged in sales or promotional materials.

The advice and strategies contained herein may not be appropriate in every situation. In selling this work, the publisher may not offer medical, legal or other professional advice or services. If professional help is needed, the services of a competent professional should be sought. Neither the publisher nor the author shall be liable for damages resulting therefrom.

The mention of a person, organization or website in this work as a potential source of quotes and/or further information does not imply that the author or publisher endorses the information that may be provided by that person, organization or website or the advice they/it may give. suggestions they/it may have made. In addition, readers should be aware that the websites listed in this work may have changed or disappeared. In addition, readers should be aware that the websites listed in this work may have changed or disappeared between the time this work was written and the time it was read.

By using this recipe book, you agree to abide by the terms outlined in this copyright statement and disclaimer.

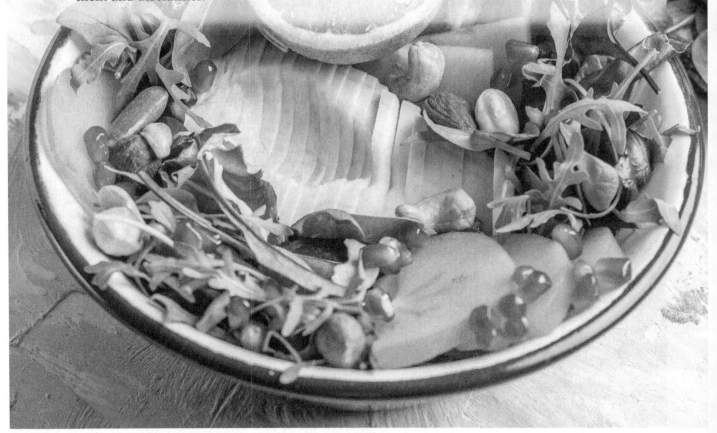

CONTENTS

37   Fish And Seafood Recipes

48   Beans , Grains, And Pastas Recipes

INTRODUCTION

Timothy R. Mooneyhan is a seasoned chef, nutritionist, and culinary explorer dedicated to promoting health and wellness through the delights of Mediterranean cuisine. With over two decades of experience in the culinary world, Tim has honed his craft in both professional kitchens and through extensive travels across Mediterranean countries.

As a certified nutritionist, Tim combines his passion for cooking with his in-depth knowledge of nutrition to create recipes that are not only delicious but also health-conscious. His commitment to helping others make positive dietary choices led him to write the "Mediterranean Diet Cookbook."

The process of writing this cookbook was a labor of love. Drawing inspiration from the vibrant markets, coastal villages, and family kitchens he encountered during his Mediterranean journeys, Tim meticulously crafted a collection of recipes that capture the essence of Mediterranean living. He collaborated with local chefs and home cooks, delving into regional traditions and ingredients to create a diverse and authentic culinary experience for his readers.

Tim's mission with the "Mediterranean Diet Cookbook" goes beyond providing recipes; it's about sharing a way of life. He believes in the transformative power of food and its ability to foster not only physical health but also cultural appreciation and a deeper connection to one's own well-being.

When he's not in the kitchen or writing, Tim enjoys educating others about the Mediterranean lifestyle through cooking classes, workshops, and wellness seminars. His enthusiasm for the Mediterranean way of life shines through in every page of his cookbook, making it not just a collection of recipes but a journey of discovery, health, and gastronomic pleasure.

Timothy R. Mooneyhan's "Mediterranean Diet Cookbook" is a testament to his dedication to helping individuals savor the flavors of the Mediterranean while nurturing their bodies and spirits. With his cookbook in hand, readers can embark on a culinary adventure that promotes longevity, well-being, and a profound appreciation for the art of Mediterranean cooking.

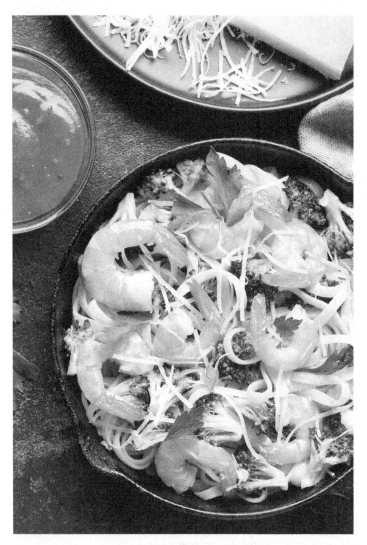

ORIGIN OF THE MEDITER-RANEAN DIET

The Mediterranean Diet has ancient origins rooted in the dietary habits of civilizations bordering the Mediterranean Sea. Dating back thousands of years, this dietary pattern is deeply entwined with the agricultural traditions of the region, emphasizing the consumption of locally sourced fruits, vegetables, whole grains, and legumes. Seafood, notably fish, was a prominent source of protein, and olive oil was a key dietary fat. The diet's cultural significance lies in its communal approach to meals and the leisurely enjoyment of fresh, seasonal ingredients. It represents a historical way of life, reflecting the availability of abundant, nutrient-rich foods and fostering a profound connection between people, their environment, and their culinary heritage.

KEY COMPONENTS: THE DIET'S CORE COMPONENTS INCLUDE:

1. High consumption of fruits and vegetables.

2. Whole grains like wheat, rice, and oats.

3. Healthy fats, mainly from olive oil and nuts.

4. Lean protein sources, such as fish and poultry.

5. Moderate consumption of dairy products, primarily yogurt and cheese.

6. Limited red meat intake.

7. Red wine in moderation, usually consumed with meals.

THE MEDITERRANEAN DIET PYRAMID

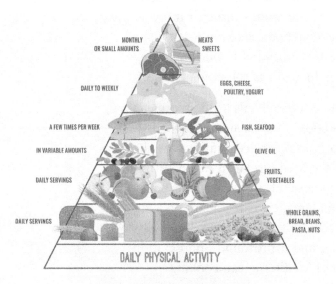

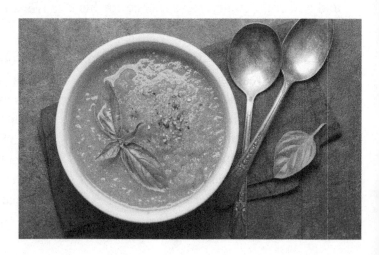

PEOPLE ON THE MEDITERRANEAN DIET

Individuals of All Ages: The Mediterranean Diet is suitable for people of all ages, from children to seniors. It can support the nutritional needs and overall health of individuals at different life stages.

Health-Conscious Individuals: People who prioritize their health and well-being can benefit from the Mediterranean Diet. It is associated with a reduced risk of chronic diseases such as heart disease, diabetes, and certain cancers.

Weight Management: The Mediterranean Diet can be an excellent choice for those looking to manage or maintain a healthy weight. It emphasizes whole, nutrient-dense foods and portion control.

Heart Health: Individuals with a focus on heart health, especially those with a family history of cardiovascular issues, can find the Mediterranean Diet particularly beneficial due to its emphasis on healthy fats, such as those from olive oil, and its potential to lower cholesterol levels.

Vegetarians and Vegans: The Mediterranean Diet is adaptable to various dietary preferences. Vegetarians can enjoy the plant-based aspects, while vegans can exclude animal products and still follow the diet's principles with plant-based sources of protein.

Diabetics: The Mediterranean Diet's emphasis on whole grains, legumes, and lean proteins can be suitable for individuals with diabetes, as it may help stabilize blood sugar levels.

Food Enthusiasts: Those who appreciate delicious, flavorful cuisine will find the Mediterranean Diet appealing. It features a variety of herbs, spices, and seasonings that enhance the taste of dishes.

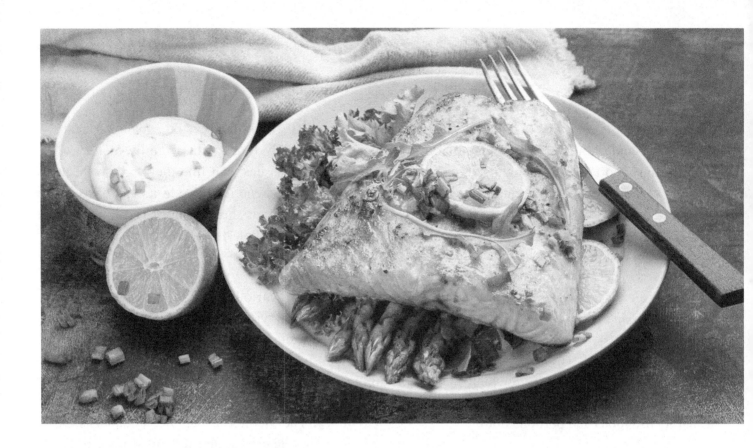

HOW TO INTEGRATE THE MEDITERRANEAN LIFE-STYLE INTO YOUR LIFE?

Incorporating the Mediterranean lifestyle into your life involves adopting not just a dietary pattern but also a holistic approach to well-being and living.

Adopt Mediterranean Meal Patterns:

1. Share Meals: Cultivate a sense of community by enjoying meals with family and friends. Make mealtime a social and enjoyable experience.

2. Mindful Eating: Savor your food slowly, paying attention to flavors and textures. Avoid distractions like TV or smartphones during meals.

3. Smaller Portions: Practice portion control to avoid overeating. Serve smaller servings and have seconds if needed.

4. Cook at Home: Prepare homemade meals using fresh ingredients whenever possible. Cooking at home allows you to have better control over what you eat.

5. Stay Physically Active:Incorporate Regular Exercise: Engage in physical activity regularly, aiming for at least 30 minutes of moderate exercise most days of the week. Activities like walking, swimming, and cycling are great choices.

6. Stay Hydrated:Water is the preferred beverage. Keep well-hydrated throughout the day.

7. Manage Stress:Mediterranean living emphasizes a relaxed pace of life. Find stress-relief techniques that work for you, such as meditation, yoga, or spending time in nature.

8. Get Sufficient Rest:Aim for 7-9 hours of quality sleep each night to promote overall well-being.

REASONS FOR MEDITERRANEAN DIET COOKBOOK

HEALTH BENEFITS

The Mediterranean Diet is well-documented for its numerous health benefits. Recommending a recipe book allows individuals to easily access and incorporate these health-promoting foods into their daily meals. It can help reduce the risk of chronic diseases such as heart disease, diabetes, and certain cancers.

DIVERSE AND DELICIOUS MEALS

A Mediterranean Diet recipe book offers a wide variety of flavorful and satisfying recipes. It introduces individuals to new ingredients, flavors, and cooking techniques, making healthy eating enjoyable and sustainable.

BALANCED APPROACH

The diet promotes a balanced approach to nutrition, emphasizing the importance of portion control and moderation. A recipe book provides guidance on portion sizes and meal planning, helping individuals maintain a healthy weight.

EASY AND ACCESSIBLE

Recipe books offer step-by-step instructions and cooking tips, making it easier for both beginners and experienced cooks to prepare Mediterranean-style meals. They provide accessible guidance for incorporating this dietary pattern into daily life.

WEIGHT MANAGEMENT

For those looking to manage their weight, a Mediterranean Diet recipe book provides recipes and meal plans that support healthy weight loss and maintenance goals.

LONGEVITY AND WELL-BEING

The Mediterranean Diet is associated with increased longevity and overall well-being. Recommending a recipe book encourages individuals to adopt a dietary pattern that supports a healthier, more vibrant life.

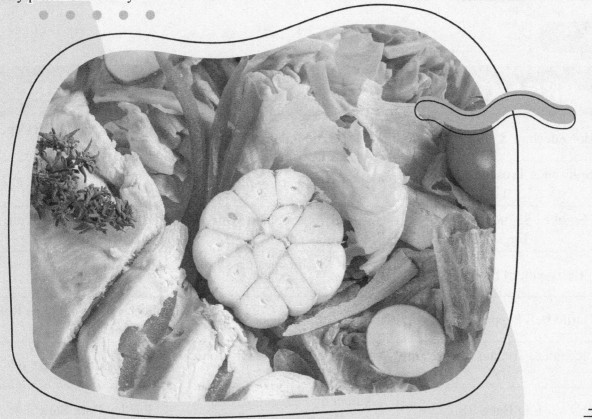

4 -WEEK Meal Plans

WEEK 1

DAY	BREAKFAST	LUNCH	DINNER
1	Apple & Date Smoothie 15	Ricotta & Olive Rigatoni 49	Italian Potato & Chicken 61
2	Eggs Florentine With Pancetta 15	Arrabbiata Penne Rigate 49	Balsamic Chicken Breasts With Feta 61
3	Ricotta Toast With Strawberries 15	Bulgur Pilaf With Garbanzo 49	Rich Pork In Cilantro Sauce 61
4	Feta And Spinach Frittata 16	Rigatoni With Peppers & Mozzarella 49	Rosemary Tomato Chicken 61
5	Falafel Balls With Tahini Sauce 16	Vegetable Lentils With Brown Rice 50	Baked Chicken & Veggie 62
6	Healthy Chia Pudding 15	Tomato Sauce And Basil Pesto Fettuccine 50	Cilantro Turkey Penne With Asparagus 62
7	Tomato And Egg Scramble 17	Roasted Butternut Squash And Zucchini With Penne 50	Provençal Flank Steak Au Pistou 62

WEEK 2

DAY	BREAKFAST	LUNCH	DINNER
1	Hot Zucchini & Egg Nests 17	Classic Falafel 51	Paprika Chicken With Caper Dressing 62
2	Spinach & Prosciutto Crostini 17	Mediterranean Lentils 51	Sweet Chicken Stew 63
3	Smoked Salmon Scrambled Eggs 17	Rice & Lentil Salad With Caramelized Onions 52	Slow Cooker Beef With Tomatoes 63
4	Berry-yogurt Smoothie 18	Eggplant & Chickpea Casserole 52	Chermoula Roasted Pork Tenderloin 63
5	Garlic Bell Pepper Omelet 19	Ribollita (tuscan Bean Soup) 52	Spinach-ricotta Chicken Rolls 63
6	Zucchini & Tomato Cheese Tart 18	Autumn Vegetable & Rigatoni Bake 52	Date Lamb Tangine 64
7	Egg Bake 18	Authentic Fettuccine A La Puttanesca 53	Parsley Pork Stew 64

WEEK 3

DAY	BREAKFAST	LUNCH	DINNER
1	Marinara Poached Eggs 19	Swoodles With Almond Butter Sauce 53	Parsley-dijon Chicken And Potatoes 64
2	Pecorino Bulgur & Spinach Cupcakes 19	Freekeh Pilaf With Dates And Pistachios 53	Greek-style Chicken With Potatoes 64
3	Berry And Nut Parfait 19	Mozzarella & Asparagus Pasta 54	Chicken Drumsticks With Peach Glaze 65
4	Almond Iced-coffee 20	Spaghetti With Pine Nuts And Cheese 54	Honey Mustard Pork Chops 65
5	Parmesan Oatmeal With Greens 20	Genovese Mussel Linguine 54	Juicy Pork Chops 65
6	Easy Buckwheat Porridge 20	Cumin Quinoa Pilaf 55	Marsala Chicken With Mushrooms 66
7	Avocado And Egg Toast 21	Valencian-style Mussel Rice 55	Pork Chops In Wine Sauce 66

WEEK 4

DAY	BREAKFAST	LUNCH	DINNER
1	Yummy Lentil Stuffed Pitas 21	Slow Cooked Turkey And Brown Rice 55	Tomato Walnut Chicken 66
2	Breakfast Shakshuka Bake 21	Marrakech-style Couscous 56	Greek-style Veggie & Beef In Pita 66
3	Brown Rice And Black Bean Burgers 22	Bulgur Pilaf With Kale And Tomatoes 56	Herby Chicken With Asparagus Sauce 67
4	Carrot & Pecan Cupcakes 22	Brown Rice Pilaf With Pistachios And Raisins 56	Garlicky Beef With Walnuts 67
5	Mediterranean Omelet 23	Spinach & Salmon Fettuccine In White Sauce 56	Easy Pork Stew 67
6	Greek Vegetable Salad Pita 23	Mustard Vegetable Millet 57	Potato Lamb And Olive Stew 68
7	Veg Mix And Blackeye Pea Burritos 24	Cheesy Sage Farro 57	French Chicken Cassoulet 68

BREAKFAST RECIPES

Apple & Date Smoothie

Servings:1
Cooking Time:5 Minutes

Ingredients:
- 1 apple, peeled and chopped
- ½ cup milk
- 4 dates
- 1 tsp ground cinnamon

Directions:
1. In a blender, place the milk, ½ cup of water, dates, cinnamon, and apple. Blitz until smooth. Let chill in the fridge for 30 minutes. Serve in a tall glass.

Nutrition Info:
- Per Serving: Calories: 486;Fat: 29g;Protein: 4.2g;Carbs: 63g.

Eggs Florentine With Pancetta

Servings:2
Cooking Time:20 Minutes

Ingredients:
- 1 English muffin, toasted and halved
- ¼ cup chopped pancetta
- 2 tsp hollandaise sauce
- 1 cup spinach
- Salt and black pepper to taste
- 2 large eggs

Directions:
1. Place pancetta in a pan over medium heat and cook for 5 minutes until crispy; reserve. Add the baby spinach and cook for 2-3 minutes in the same pan until the spinach wilts. Fill a pot with 3 inches of water over medium heat and bring to a boil. Add 1 tbsp of vinegar and reduce the heat.
2. Crack the eggs one at a time into a small dish and gently pour into the simmering water. Poach the eggs for 2-3 minutes until the whites are set, but the yolks are still soft; remove with a slotted spoon. Divide the spinach between muffin halves and top with pancetta and poached eggs. Spoon the hollandaise sauce on top and serve.

Nutrition Info:
- Per Serving: Calories: 173;Fat: 7g;Protein: 11g;Carbs: 17g.

Ricotta Toast With Strawberries

Servings:2
Cooking Time: 0 Minutes

Ingredients:
- ½ cup crumbled ricotta cheese
- 1 tablespoon honey, plus additional as needed
- Pinch of sea salt, plus additional as needed
- 4 slices of whole-grain bread, toasted
- 1 cup sliced fresh strawberries
- 4 large fresh basil leaves, sliced into thin shreds

Directions:
1. Mix together the cheese, honey, and salt in a small bowl until well incorporated.
2. Taste and add additional salt and honey if needed.
3. Spoon 2 tablespoons of the cheese mixture onto each slice of bread and spread it all over.
4. Sprinkle the sliced strawberry and basil leaves on top before serving.

Nutrition Info:
- Per Serving: Calories: 274;Fat: 7.9g;Protein: 15.1g;-Carbs: 39.8g.

Healthy Chia Pudding

Servings:4
Cooking Time: 0 Minutes

Ingredients:
- 4 cups unsweetened almond milk
- ¾ cup chia seeds
- 1 teaspoon ground cinnamon
- Pinch sea salt

Directions:
1. In a medium bowl, whisk together the almond milk, chia seeds, cinnamon, and sea salt until well incorporated.
2. Cover and transfer to the refrigerator to thicken for about 1 hour, or until a pudding-like texture is achieved.
3. Serve chilled.

Nutrition Info:
- Per Serving: Calories: 236;Fat: 9.8g;Protein: 13.1g;-Carbs: 24.8g.

Falafel Balls With Tahini Sauce

Servings:4
Cooking Time: 20 Minutes

Ingredients:
- Tahini Sauce:
- ½ cup tahini
- 2 tablespoons lemon juice
- ¼ cup finely chopped flat-leaf parsley
- 2 cloves garlic, minced
- ½ cup cold water, as needed
- Falafel:
- 1 cup dried chickpeas, soaked overnight, drained
- ¼ cup chopped flat-leaf parsley
- ¼ cup chopped cilantro
- 1 large onion, chopped
- 1 teaspoon cumin
- ½ teaspoon chili flakes
- 4 cloves garlic
- 1 teaspoon sea salt
- 5 tablespoons almond flour
- 1½ teaspoons baking soda, dissolved in 1 teaspoon water
- 2 cups peanut oil
- 1 medium bell pepper, chopped
- 1 medium tomato, chopped
- 4 whole-wheat pita breads

Directions:
1. Make the Tahini Sauce:
2. Combine the ingredients for the tahini sauce in a small bowl. Stir to mix well until smooth.
3. Wrap the bowl in plastic and refrigerate until ready to serve.
4. Make the Falafel:
5. Put the chickpeas, parsley, cilantro, onion, cumin, chili flakes, garlic, and salt in a food processor. Pulse to mix well but not puréed.
6. Add the flour and baking soda to the food processor, then pulse to form a smooth and tight dough.
7. Put the dough in a large bowl and wrap in plastic. Refrigerate for at least 2 hours to let it rise.
8. Divide and shape the dough into walnut-sized small balls.
9. Pour the peanut oil in a large pot and heat over high heat until the temperature of the oil reaches 375ºF.
10. Drop 6 balls into the oil each time, and fry for 5 minutes or until golden brown and crispy. Turn the balls with a strainer to make them fried evenly.
11. Transfer the balls on paper towels with the strainer, then drain the oil from the balls.
12. Roast the pita breads in the oven for 5 minutes or until golden brown, if needed, then stuff the pitas with falafel balls and top with bell peppers and tomatoes. Drizzle with tahini sauce and serve immediately.

Nutrition Info:
- Per Serving: Calories: 574;Fat: 27.1g;Protein: 19.8g;- Carbs: 69.7g.

Feta And Spinach Frittata

Servings:2
Cooking Time: 15 Minutes

Ingredients:
- 4 large eggs, beaten
- 2 tablespoons fresh chopped herbs, such as rosemary, thyme, oregano, basil or 1 teaspoon dried herbs
- ¼ teaspoon salt
- Freshly ground black pepper, to taste
- 4 tablespoons extra-virgin olive oil, divided
- 1 cup fresh spinach, arugula, kale, or other leafy greens
- 4 ounces quartered artichoke hearts, rinsed, drained, and thoroughly dried
- 8 cherry tomatoes, halved
- ½ cup crumbled soft goat cheese

Directions:
1. Preheat the broiler to Low.
2. In a small bowl, combine the beaten eggs, herbs, salt, and pepper and whisk well with a fork. Set aside.
3. In an ovenproof skillet, heat 2 tablespoons of olive oil over medium heat. Add the spinach, artichoke hearts, and cherry tomatoes and sauté until just wilted, 1 to 2 minutes.
4. Pour in the egg mixture and let it cook undisturbed over medium heat for 3 to 4 minutes, until the eggs begin to set on the bottom.
5. Sprinkle the goat cheese across the top of the egg mixture and transfer the skillet to the oven.
6. Broil for 4 to 5 minutes, or until the frittata is firm in the center and golden brown on top.
7. Remove from the oven and run a rubber spatula around the edge to loosen the sides. Slice the frittata in half and serve drizzled with the remaining 2 tablespoons of olive oil.

Nutrition Info:
- Per Serving: Calories: 529;Fat: 46.5g;Protein: 21.4g;- Carbs: 7.1g.

Tomato And Egg Scramble

Servings:4
Cooking Time: 20 Minutes

Ingredients:
- 2 tablespoons extra-virgin olive oil
- ¼ cup finely minced red onion
- 1½ cups chopped fresh tomatoes
- 2 garlic cloves, minced
- ½ teaspoon dried thyme
- ½ teaspoon dried oregano
- 8 large eggs
- ½ teaspoon salt
- ¼ teaspoon freshly ground black pepper
- ¾ cup crumbled feta cheese
- ¼ cup chopped fresh mint leaves

Directions:
1. Heat the olive oil in a large skillet over medium heat.
2. Sauté the red onion and tomatoes in the hot skillet for 10 to 12 minutes, or until the tomatoes are softened.
3. Stir in the garlic, thyme, and oregano and sauté for 2 to 4 minutes, or until the garlic is fragrant.
4. Meanwhile, beat the eggs with the salt and pepper in a medium bowl until frothy.
5. Pour the beaten eggs into the skillet and reduce the heat to low. Scramble
6. for 3 to 4 minutes, stirring constantly, or until the eggs are set.
7. Remove from the heat and scatter with the feta cheese and mint. Serve warm.

Nutrition Info:
- Per Serving: Calories: 260;Fat: 21.9g;Protein: 10.2g;-Carbs: 5.8g.

Hot Zucchini & Egg Nests

Servings:4
Cooking Time:25 Minutes

Ingredients:
- 2 tbsp olive oil
- 4 eggs
- 1 lb zucchinis, shredded
- Salt and black pepper to taste
- ½ red chili pepper, minced
- 2 tbsp parsley, chopped

Directions:
1. Preheat the oven to 360 F. Combine zucchini, salt, pepper, and olive oil in a bowl. Form nest shapes with a spoon onto a greased baking sheet. Crack an egg into each nest and season with salt, pepper, and chili pepper. Bake for 11 minutes. Serve topped with parsley.

Nutrition Info:
- Per Serving: Calories: 141;Fat: 11.6g;Protein: 7g;Carbs: 4.2g.

Spinach & Prosciutto Crostini

Servings:1
Cooking Time:5 Minutes

Ingredients:
- 1 tsp olive oil
- 2 prosciutto slices
- 2 ciabatta slices, toasted
- 1 tbsp Dijon mustard
- Salt and black pepper to taste
- 1 tomato, sliced
- ¼ cup baby spinach

Directions:
1. Smear Dijon mustard on one side of each ciabatta slice and top with prosciutto, tomato, spinach, salt, and pepper on each slice. Drizzle with olive oil and serve.

Nutrition Info:
- Per Serving: Calories: 250;Fat: 12g;Protein: 9g;Carbs: 18g.

Smoked Salmon Scrambled Eggs

Servings:4
Cooking Time:15 Minutes

Ingredients:
- 2 tbsp olive oil
- 4 oz smoked salmon, flaked
- ½ red onion, finely chopped
- 8 eggs
- Salt and black pepper to taste
- ½ tsp garlic powder
- 1 scallion, chopped
- 2 tbsp green olives, chopped

Directions:
1. Beat eggs, garlic powder, salt, and pepper in a bowl. Warm olive oil in a skillet over medium heat. Stir in onion and sauté for 1-2 minutes. Add in olives and salmon and cook for another minute. Pour in the eggs and stir-fry for 5-6 minutes until the eggs are set. Serve topped with scallion.

Nutrition Info:
- Per Serving: Calories: 233;Fat: 17.5g;Protein: 18g;Carbs: 3g.

Berry-yogurt Smoothie

Servings:1
Cooking Time:5 Minutes

Ingredients:
- ½ cup Greek yogurt
- ¼ cup milk
- ½ cup fresh blueberries
- 1 tsp vanilla sugar
- 2 ice cubes

Directions:
1. Pulse the Greek yogurt, milk, vanilla sugar, and berries in your blender until the berries are liquefied. Add the ice cubes and blend on high until thick and smooth. Serve.

Nutrition Info:
- Per Serving: Calories: 230;Fat: 8.8g;Protein: 16g;Carbs: 23g.

Egg Bake

Servings:2
Cooking Time: 30 Minutes

Ingredients:
- 1 tablespoon olive oil
- 1 slice whole-grain bread
- 4 large eggs
- 3 tablespoons unsweetened almond milk
- ½ teaspoon onion powder
- ¼ teaspoon garlic powder
- ¾ cup chopped cherry tomatoes
- ¼ teaspoon salt
- Pinch freshly ground black pepper

Directions:
1. Preheat the oven to 375ºF.
2. Coat two ramekins with the olive oil and transfer to a baking sheet. Line the bottom of each ramekin with ½ of bread slice.
3. In a medium bowl, whisk together the eggs, almond milk, onion powder, garlic powder, tomatoes, salt, and pepper until well combined.
4. Pour the mixture evenly into two ramekins. Bake in the preheated oven for 30 minutes, or until the eggs are completely set.
5. Cool for 5 minutes before serving.

Nutrition Info:
- Per Serving: Calories: 240;Fat: 17.4g;Protein: 9.0g;-Carbs: 12.2g.

Zucchini & Tomato Cheese Tart

Servings:6
Cooking Time:60 Minutes

Ingredients:
- 3 tbsp olive oil
- 5 sun-dried tomatoes, chopped
- 1 prepared pie crust
- 1 onion, chopped
- 2 garlic cloves, minced
- 2 zucchinis, chopped
- 1 red bell pepper, chopped
- 6 Kalamata olives, sliced
- 1 tsp fresh dill, chopped
- ½ cup Greek yogurt
- 1 cup feta cheese, crumbled
- 4 eggs
- 1 ½ cups milk
- Salt and black pepper to taste

Directions:
1. Preheat the oven to 380 F. Warm the olive oil in a skillet over medium heat and sauté garlic and onion for 3 minutes. Add in bell pepper and zucchini and sauté for another 3 minutes. Stir in olives, dill, salt, and pepper for 1-2 minutes and add tomatoes and feta cheese. Mix well and turn the heat off.
2. Press the crust gently into a lightly greased pie dish and prick it with a fork. Bake in the oven for 10-15 minutes until pale gold. Spread the zucchini mixture over the pie crust. Whisk the eggs with salt, pepper, milk, and yogurt in a bowl, then pour over the zucchini layer. Bake for 25-30 minutes until golden brown. Let cool before serving.

Nutrition Info:
- Per Serving: Calories: 220;Fat: 16g;Protein: 10g;Carbs: 14g.

Garlic Bell Pepper Omelet

Servings:2
Cooking Time:10 Minutes

Ingredients:

- 2 tbsp olive oil
- 2 red bell peppers, chopped
- ¼ tsp nutmeg
- 4 eggs, beaten
- 2 garlic cloves, crushed
- 1 tsp Italian seasoning

Directions:

1. Heat the oil in a skillet over medium heat. Stir-fry the peppers for 3 minutes or until lightly charred; reserve. Add the garlic to the skillet and sauté for 1 minute. Pour the eggs over the garlic, sprinkle with Italian seasoning and nutmeg, and cook for 2-3 minutes or until set. Using a spatula, loosen the edges and gently slide onto a plate. Add charred peppers and fold over. Serve hot.

Nutrition Info:

- Per Serving: Calories: 272;Fat: 22g;Protein: 12g;Carbs: 6.4g.

Marinara Poached Eggs

Servings:6
Cooking Time: 15 Minutes

Ingredients:

- 1 tablespoon extra-virgin olive oil
- 1 cup chopped onion
- 2 garlic cloves, minced
- 2 cans no-salt-added Italian diced tomatoes, undrained
- 6 large eggs
- ½ cup chopped fresh flat-leaf parsley

Directions:

1. Heat the olive oil in a large skillet over medium-high heat.
2. Add the onion and sauté for 5 minutes, stirring occasionally. Add the garlic and cook for 1 minute more.
3. Pour the tomatoes with their juices over the onion mixture and cook for 2 to 3 minutes until bubbling.
4. Reduce the heat to medium and use a large spoon to make six indentations in the tomato mixture. Crack the eggs, one at a time, into each indentation.
5. Cover and simmer for 6 to 7 minutes, or until the eggs are cooked to your preference.
6. Serve with the parsley sprinkled on top.

Nutrition Info:

- Per Serving: Calories: 89;Fat: 6.0g;Protein: 4.0g;Carbs: 4.0g.

Pecorino Bulgur & Spinach Cupcakes

Servings:6
Cooking Time:45 Minutes

Ingredients:

- 2 eggs, whisked
- 1 cup bulgur
- 3 cups water
- 1 cup spinach, torn
- 2 spring onions, chopped
- ¼ cup Pecorino cheese, grated
- ½ tsp garlic powder
- Sea salt and pepper to taste
- ½ tsp dried oregano

Directions:

1. Preheat the oven to 340 F. Grease a muffin tin with cooking spray. Warm 2 cups of salted water in a saucepan over medium heat and add in bulgur. Bring to a boil and cook for 10-15 minutes. Remove to a bowl and fluff with a fork. Stir in spinach, spring onions, eggs, Pecorino cheese, garlic powder, salt, pepper, and oregano. Divide between muffin holes and bake for 25 minutes. Serve chilled.

Nutrition Info:

- Per Serving: Calories: 280;Fat: 12g;Protein: 5g;Carbs: 9g.

Berry And Nut Parfait

Servings:2
Cooking Time: 0 Minutes

Ingredients:

- 2 cups plain Greek yogurt
- 2 tablespoons honey
- 1 cup fresh raspberries
- 1 cup fresh blueberries
- ½ cup walnut pieces

Directions:

1. In a medium bowl, whisk the yogurt and honey. Spoon into 2 serving bowls.
2. Top each with ½ cup blueberries, ½ cup raspberries, and ¼ cup walnut pieces. Serve immediately.

Nutrition Info:

- Per Serving: Calories: 507;Fat: 23.0g;Protein: 24.1g;-Carbs: 57.0g.

Almond Iced-coffee

Servings:1
Cooking Time:5 Minutes

Ingredients:
- 1 cup brewed black coffee, warm
- 1 tbsp olive oil
- 1 tsp MCT oil
- 1 tbsp heavy cream
- ½ tsp almond extract
- ½ tsp ground cinnamon

Directions:
1. Pour the warm coffee (not hot) into a blender. Add the olive oil, heavy cream, MCT oil, almond extract, and cinnamon. Blend well until smooth and creamy. Drink warm and enjoy.

Nutrition Info:
- Per Serving: Calories: 128;Fat: 14.2g;Protein: 0g;Carbs: 0g.

Parmesan Oatmeal With Greens

Servings:2
Cooking Time: 18 Minutes

Ingredients:
- 1 tablespoon olive oil
- ¼ cup minced onion
- 2 cups greens (arugula, baby spinach, chopped kale, or Swiss chard)
- ¾ cup gluten-free old-fashioned oats
- 1½ cups water, or low-sodium chicken stock
- 2 tablespoons Parmesan cheese
- Salt, to taste
- Pinch freshly ground black pepper

Directions:
1. Heat the olive oil in a saucepan over medium-high heat. Add the minced onion and sauté for 2 minutes, or until softened.
2. Add the greens and stir until they begin to wilt. Transfer this mixture to a bowl and set aside.
3. Add the oats to the pan and let them toast for about 2 minutes. Add the water and bring the oats to a boil.
4. Reduce the heat to low, cover, and let the oats cook for 10 minutes, or until the liquid is absorbed and the oats are tender.
5. Stir the Parmesan cheese into the oats, and add the onion and greens back to the pan. Add additional water if needed, so the oats are creamy and not dry.
6. Stir well and season with salt and black pepper to taste. Serve warm.

Nutrition Info:
- Per Serving: Calories: 257;Fat: 14.0g;Protein: 12.2g;-

Carbs: 30.2g.

Easy Buckwheat Porridge

Servings:4
Cooking Time: 40 Minutes

Ingredients:
- 3 cups water
- 2 cups raw buckwheat groats
- Pinch sea salt
- 1 cup unsweetened almond milk

Directions:
1. In a medium saucepan, add the water, buckwheat groats, and sea salt and bring to a boil over medium-high heat.
2. Once it starts to boil, reduce the heat to low. Cook for about 20 minutes, stirring occasionally, or until most of the water is absorbed.
3. Fold in the almond milk and whisk well. Continue cooking for about 15 minutes, or until the buckwheat groats are very softened.
4. Ladle the porridge into bowls and serve warm.

Nutrition Info:
- Per Serving: Calories: 121;Fat: 1.0g;Protein: 6.3g;Carbs: 21.5g.

Cinnamon Oatmeal With Dried Cranberries

Servings:2
Cooking Time: 8 Minutes

Ingredients:
- 1 cup almond milk
- 1 cup water
- Pinch sea salt
- 1 cup old-fashioned oats
- ½ cup dried cranberries
- 1 teaspoon ground cinnamon

Directions:
1. In a medium saucepan over high heat, bring the almond milk, water, and salt to a boil.
2. Stir in the oats, cranberries, and cinnamon. Reduce the heat to medium and cook for 5 minutes, stirring occasionally.
3. Remove the oatmeal from the heat. Cover and let it stand for 3 minutes. Stir before serving.

Nutrition Info:
- Per Serving: Calories: 107;Fat: 2.1g;Protein: 3.2g;Carbs: 18.2g.

Avocado And Egg Toast

Servings:2
Cooking Time: 8 Minutes

Ingredients:

- 2 tablespoons ground flaxseed
- ½ teaspoon baking powder
- 2 large eggs, beaten
- 1 teaspoon salt, plus additional for serving
- ½ teaspoon freshly ground black pepper, plus additional for serving
- ½ teaspoon garlic powder, sesame seed, caraway seed, or other dried herbs (optional)
- 3 tablespoons extra-virgin olive oil, divided
- 1 medium ripe avocado, peeled, pitted, and sliced
- 2 tablespoons chopped ripe tomato

Directions:

1. In a small bowl, combine the flaxseed and baking powder, breaking up any lumps in the baking powder.
2. Add the beaten eggs, salt, pepper, and garlic powder (if desired) and whisk well. Let sit for 2 minutes.
3. In a small nonstick skillet, heat 1 tablespoon of olive oil over medium heat. Pour the egg mixture into the skillet and let cook undisturbed until the egg begins to set on bottom, 2 to 3 minutes.
4. Using a rubber spatula, scrape down the sides to allow uncooked egg to reach the bottom. Cook for an additional 2 to 3 minutes.
5. Once almost set, flip like a pancake and allow the top to fully cook, another 1 to 2 minutes.
6. Remove from the skillet and allow to cool slightly, then slice into 2 pieces.
7. Top each piece with avocado slices, additional salt and pepper, chopped tomato, and drizzle with the remaining 2 tablespoons of olive oil. Serve immediately.

Nutrition Info:

- Per Serving: Calories: 297;Fat: 26.1g;Protein: 8.9g;-Carbs: 12.0g.

Yummy Lentil Stuffed Pitas

Servings:4
Cooking Time:20 Minutes

Ingredients:

- 4 pitta breads, halved horizontally
- 2 tbsp olive oil
- 1 tomato, cubed
- 1 red onion, chopped
- 1 garlic clove, minced
- ¼ cup parsley, chopped
- 1 cup lentils, rinsed
- ¼ cup lemon juice
- Salt and black pepper to taste

Directions:

1. Bring a pot of salted water to a boil over high heat. Pour in the lentils and lower the heat. Cover and let it simmer for 15 minutes or until lentils are tender, adding more water if needed. Drain and set aside.
2. Warm the olive oil in a skillet over medium heat and cook the onion and garlic and for 3 minutes until soft and translucent. Stir in tomato, lemon juice, salt, and pepper and cook for another 10 minutes. Add the lentils and parsley to the skillet and stir to combine. Fill the pita bread with the lentil mixture. Roll up and serve immediately. Enjoy!

Nutrition Info:

- Per Serving: Calories: 390;Fat: 2g;Protein: 29g;Carbs: 68g.

Breakfast Shakshuka Bake

Servings:4
Cooking Time:25 Minutes

Ingredients:

- 2 tbsp extra-virgin olive oil
- 1 cup chopped red onion
- 1 chopped red bell pepper
- 1 cup finely diced potatoes
- 1 tsp garlic powder
- 1 can diced tomatoes
- ¼ tsp turmeric
- ¼ tsp paprika
- ¼ tsp dried oregano
- ¼ tsp ground cardamom
- 4 large eggs
- ¼ cup chopped fresh cilantro

Directions:

1. Preheat oven to 350 F. Warn the olive oil in a skillet over medium heat and sauté the shallots for about 3 minutes, until fragrant. Add bell peppers, potatoes, oregano, and garlic powder. Cook for 10 minutes, stirring often.
2. Pour in the tomatoes, turmeric, paprika, and cardamom and mix well until bubbly. Heat off. With a wooden spoon, make 4 holes in the mixture and crack the eggs into each space.
3. Put the skillet in the oven and cook for an additional 5-10 minutes until the whites are set, but the yolk is still runny. Sprinkle with the cilantro and serve.

Nutrition Info:

- Per Serving: Calories: 224;Fat: 12g;Protein: 9g;Carbs: 19.7g.

Brown Rice And Black Bean Burgers

Servings:8
Cooking Time: 40 Minutes

Ingredients:

- 1 cup cooked brown rice
- 1 can black beans, drained and rinsed
- 1 tablespoon olive oil
- 2 tablespoons taco or seasoning
- ½ yellow onion, finely diced
- 1 beet, peeled and grated
- 1 carrot, peeled and grated
- 2 tablespoons no-salt-added tomato paste
- 2 tablespoons apple cider vinegar
- 3 garlic cloves, minced
- ¼ teaspoon sea salt
- Ground black pepper, to taste
- 8 whole-wheat hamburger buns
- Toppings:
- 16 lettuce leaves, rinsed well
- 8 tomato slices, rinsed well
- Whole-grain mustard, to taste

Directions:

1. Line a baking sheet with parchment paper.
2. Put the brown rice and black beans in a food processor and pulse until mix well. Pour the mixture in a large bowl and set aside.
3. Heat the olive oil in a nonstick skillet over medium heat until shimmering.
4. Add the taco seasoning and stir for 1 minute or until fragrant.
5. Add the onion, beet, and carrot and sauté for 5 minutes or until the onion is translucent and beet and carrot are tender.
6. Pour in the tomato paste and vinegar, then add the garlic and cook for 3 minutes or until the sauce is thickened. Sprinkle with salt and ground black pepper.
7. Transfer the vegetable mixture to the bowl of rice mixture, then stir to mix well until smooth.
8. Divide and shape the mixture into 8 patties, then arrange the patties on the baking sheet and refrigerate for at least 1 hour.
9. Preheat the oven to 400ºF.
10. Remove the baking sheet from the refrigerator and allow to sit under room temperature for 10 minutes.
11. Bake in the preheated oven for 40 minutes or until golden brown on both sides. Flip the patties halfway through the cooking time.
12. Remove the patties from the oven and allow to cool for 10 minutes.
13. Assemble the buns with patties, lettuce, and tomato slices. Top the filling with mustard and serve immediately.

Nutrition Info:

- Per Serving: Calories: 544;Fat: 20.0g;Protein: 15.8g;-Carbs: 76.0g.

Carrot & Pecan Cupcakes

Servings:6
Cooking Time:30 Minutes

Ingredients:

- 2 tbsp olive oil
- 1 ½ cups grated carrots
- ¼ cup pecans, chopped
- 1 cup oat bran
- 1 cup wholewheat flour
- ½ cup all-purpose flour
- ½ cup old-fashioned oats
- 3 tbsp light brown sugar
- 1 tsp vanilla extract
- ½ lemon, zested
- 1 tsp baking powder
- 2 tsp ground cinnamon
- 2 tsp ground ginger
- ½ tsp ground nutmeg
- ¼ tsp salt
- 1¼ cups soy milk
- 2 tbsp honey
- 1 egg

Directions:

1. Preheat oven to 350 F. Mix whole-wheat flour, all-purpose flour, oat bran, oats, sugar, baking powder, cinnamon, nutmeg, ginger, and salt in a bowl; set aside.
2. Beat egg with soy milk, honey, vanilla, lemon zest, and olive oil in another bowl. Pour this mixture into the flour mixture and combine to blend, leaving some lumps. Stir in carrots and pecans. Spoon batter into greased muffin cups. Bake for about 20 minutes. Prick with a toothpick and if it comes out easily, the cakes are cooked done. Let cool and serve.

Nutrition Info:

- Per Serving: Calories: 346;Fat: 10g;Protein: 13g;Carbs: 59g.

Mediterranean Omelet

Servings:2
Cooking Time: 15 Minutes

Ingredients:
- 2 teaspoons extra-virgin olive oil, divided
- 1 garlic clove, minced
- ½ yellow bell pepper, thinly sliced
- ½ red bell pepper, thinly sliced
- ¼ cup thinly sliced red onion
- 2 tablespoons chopped fresh parsley, plus extra for garnish
- 2 tablespoons chopped fresh basil
- ½ teaspoon salt
- ½ teaspoon freshly ground black pepper
- 4 large eggs, beaten

Directions:
1. In a large, heavy skillet, heat 1 teaspoon of the olive oil over medium heat. Add the garlic, peppers, and onion to the skillet and sauté, stirring frequently, for 5 minutes.
2. Add the parsley, basil, salt, and pepper, increase the heat to medium-high, and sauté for 2 minutes. Slide the vegetable mixture onto a plate and return the skillet to the heat.
3. Heat the remaining 1 teaspoon of olive oil in the skillet and pour in the beaten eggs, tilting the pan to coat evenly. Cook the eggs just until the edges are bubbly and all but the center is dry, 3 to 5 minutes.
4. Spoon the vegetable mixture onto one-half of the omelet and use a spatula to fold the empty side over the top. Slide the omelet onto a platter or cutting board.
5. To serve, cut the omelet in half and garnish with extra fresh parsley.

Nutrition Info:
- Per Serving: Calories: 206;Fat: 14.2g;Protein: 13.7g;-Carbs: 7.2g.

Greek Vegetable Salad Pita

Servings:4
Cooking Time: 0 Minutes

Ingredients:
- ½ cup baby spinach leaves
- ½ small red onion, thinly sliced
- ½ small cucumber, deseeded and chopped
- 1 tomato, chopped
- 1 cup chopped romaine lettuce
- 1 tablespoon extra-virgin olive oil
- ½ tablespoon red wine vinegar
- 1 teaspoon Dijon mustard
- 1 tablespoon crumbled feta cheese
- Sea salt and freshly ground pepper, to taste
- 1 whole-wheat pita

Directions:

1. Combine all the ingredients, except for the pita, in a large bowl. Toss to mix well.
2. Stuff the pita with the salad, then serve immediately.

Nutrition Info:
- Per Serving: Calories: 137;Fat: 8.1g;Protein: 3.1g;Carbs: 14.3g.

Dulse, Avocado, And Tomato Pitas

Servings:4
Cooking Time: 30 Minutes

Ingredients:
- 2 teaspoons coconut oil
- ½ cup dulse, picked through and separated
- Ground black pepper, to taste
- 2 avocados, sliced
- 2 tablespoons lime juice
- ¼ cup chopped cilantro
- 2 scallions, white and light green parts, sliced
- Sea salt, to taste
- 4 whole wheat pitas, sliced in half
- 4 cups chopped romaine
- 4 plum tomatoes, sliced

Directions:
1. Heat the coconut oil in a nonstick skillet over medium heat until melted.
2. Add the dulse and sauté for 5 minutes or until crispy. Sprinkle with ground black pepper and turn off the heat. Set aside.
3. Put the avocado, lime juice, cilantro, and scallions in a food processor and sprinkle with salt and ground black pepper. Pulse to combine well until smooth.
4. Toast the pitas in a baking pan in the oven for 1 minute until soft.
5. Transfer the pitas to a clean work surface and open. Spread the avocado mixture over the pitas, then top with dulse, romaine, and tomato slices.
6. Serve immediately.

Nutrition Info:
- Per Serving: Calories: 412;Fat: 18.7g;Protein: 9.1g;-Carbs: 56.1g.

Veg Mix And Blackeye Pea Burritos

Servings:6
Cooking Time: 40 Minutes

Ingredients:
- 1 teaspoon olive oil
- 1 red onion, diced
- 2 garlic cloves, minced
- 1 zucchini, chopped
- 1 tomato, diced
- 1 bell pepper, any color, deseeded and diced
- 1 can blackeye peas
- 2 teaspoons chili powder
- Sea salt, to taste
- 6 whole-grain tortillas

Directions:
1. Preheat the oven to 325°F.
2. Heat the olive oil in a nonstick skillet over medium heat or until shimmering.
3. Add the onion and sauté for 5 minutes or until translucent.
4. Add the garlic and sauté for 30 seconds or until fragrant.
5. Add the zucchini and sauté for 5 minutes or until tender.
6. Add the tomato and bell pepper and sauté for 2 minutes or until soft.
7. Fold in the black peas and sprinkle them with chili powder and salt. Stir to mix well.
8. Place the tortillas on a clean work surface, then top them with sautéed vegetables mix.
9. Fold one ends of tortillas over the vegetable mix, then tuck and roll them into burritos.
10. Arrange the burritos in a baking dish, seam side down, then pour the juice remains in the skillet over the burritos.
11. Bake in the preheated oven for 25 minutes or until golden brown.
12. Serve immediately.

Nutrition Info:
- Per Serving: Calories: 335;Fat: 16.2g;Protein: 12.1g;-Carbs: 8.3g.

Chickpea Lettuce Wraps

Servings:2
Cooking Time: 0 Minutes

Ingredients:
- 1 can chickpeas, drained and rinsed well
- 1 celery stalk, diced
- ½ shallot, minced
- 1 green apple, cored and diced
- 3 tablespoons tahini (sesame paste)
- 2 teaspoons freshly squeezed lemon juice
- 1 teaspoon raw honey
- 1 teaspoon Dijon mustard
- Dash salt
- Filtered water, to thin
- 4 romaine lettuce leaves

Directions:
1. In a medium bowl, stir together the chickpeas, celery, shallot, apple, tahini, lemon juice, honey, mustard, and salt. If needed, add some water to thin the mixture.
2. Place the romaine lettuce leaves on a plate. Fill each with the chickpea filling, using it all. Wrap the leaves around the filling. Serve immediately.

Nutrition Info:
- Per Serving: Calories: 397;Fat: 15.1g;Protein: 15.1g;-Carbs: 53.1g.

Maple Peach Smoothie

Servings:2
Cooking Time:5 Minutes

Ingredients:
- 2 cups almond milk
- 2 cups peaches, chopped
- 1 cup crushed ice
- ½ tsp ground ginger
- 1 tbsp maple syrup

Directions:
1. In a food processor, mix milk, peaches, ice, maple syrup, and ginger until smooth. Serve.

Nutrition Info:
- Per Serving: Calories: 639;Fat: 58g;Protein: 7g;Carbs: 34.2g.

Dilly Salmon Frittata

Servings:4
Cooking Time:35 Minutes

Ingredients:
- 2 tbsp olive oil
- 1 cup cream cheese
- 1 cup smoked salmon, chopped
- 8 eggs, whisked
- 1 tsp dill, chopped
- 2 tbsp milk
- Salt and black pepper to taste

Directions:

1. Preheat oven to 360 F. In a bowl, place all the ingredients and stir to combine. Warm olive oil in a pan over medium heat and pour in the mixture. Cook until the base is set, about 3-4 minutes. Place the pan in the oven and bake until the top is golden, about 5 minutes. Serve sliced into wedges.

Nutrition Info:
- Per Serving: Calories: 418;Fat: 37g;Protein: 19.6g;Carbs: 3g.

Ricotta Muffins With Pear Glaze

Servings:4
Cooking Time:42 Minutes

Ingredients:
- 16 oz ricotta cheese
- 2 large eggs
- ¼ cup flour
- 1 tbsp sugar
- 1 tsp vanilla extract
- ¼ tsp ground nutmeg
- 1 pear, cored and diced
- 1 tbsp sugar

Directions:

1. Preheat the oven to 400 F. In a large bowl, whisk the ricotta, eggs, flour, sugar, vanilla, and nutmeg. Spoon into 4 greased ramekins. Bake for 20-25 minutes. Transfer to a wire rack to cool before unmolding.

2. Place the pear, sugar, and 2 tbsp of water in a small saucepan over low heat. Simmer for 10 minutes until slightly softened. Remove from the heat, and stir in the honey. Serve the ricotta ramekins glazed with pear sauce.

Nutrition Info:
- Per Serving: Calories: 329;Fat: 19g;Protein: 17g;Carbs: 23g.

Pesto Salami & Cheese Egg Cupcakes

Servings:6
Cooking Time:25 Minutes

Ingredients:
- ½ cup roasted red peppers, chopped
- 1 tbsp olive oil
- 5 eggs, whisked
- 4 oz Italian dry salami, sliced
- 1/3 cup spinach, chopped
- ¼ cup ricotta cheese, crumbled
- Salt and black pepper to taste
- 1 ½ tbsp basil pesto

Directions:

1. Preheat the oven to 380 F. Brush 6 ramekin cups with olive oil and line them with dry salami slices. Top with spinach, ricotta cheese, and roasted peppers. Whisk the eggs with pesto, salt, and pepper in a bowl and pour over the peppers. Bake for 15 minutes and serve warm.

Nutrition Info:
- Per Serving: Calories: 120;Fat: 8g;Protein: 10g;Carbs: 2g.

Mushroom-pesto Baked Pizza

Servings:2
Cooking Time: 15 Minutes

Ingredients:
- 1 teaspoon extra-virgin olive oil
- ½ cup sliced mushrooms
- ½ red onion, sliced
- Salt and freshly ground black pepper
- ¼ cup store-bought pesto sauce
- 2 whole-wheat flatbreads
- ¼ cup shredded Mozzarella cheese

Directions:

1. Preheat the oven to 350°F.
2. In a small skillet, heat the oil over medium heat. Add the mushrooms and onion, and season with salt and pepper. Sauté for 3 to 5 minutes until the onion and mushrooms begin to soften.
3. Spread 2 tablespoons of pesto on each flatbread.
4. Divide the mushroom-onion mixture between the two flatbreads. Top each with 2 tablespoons of cheese.
5. Place the flatbreads on a baking sheet and bake for 10 to 12 minutes until the cheese is melted and bubbly. Serve warm.

Nutrition Info:
- Per Serving: Calories: 348;Fat: 23.5g;Protein: 14.2g;-Carbs: 28.1g.

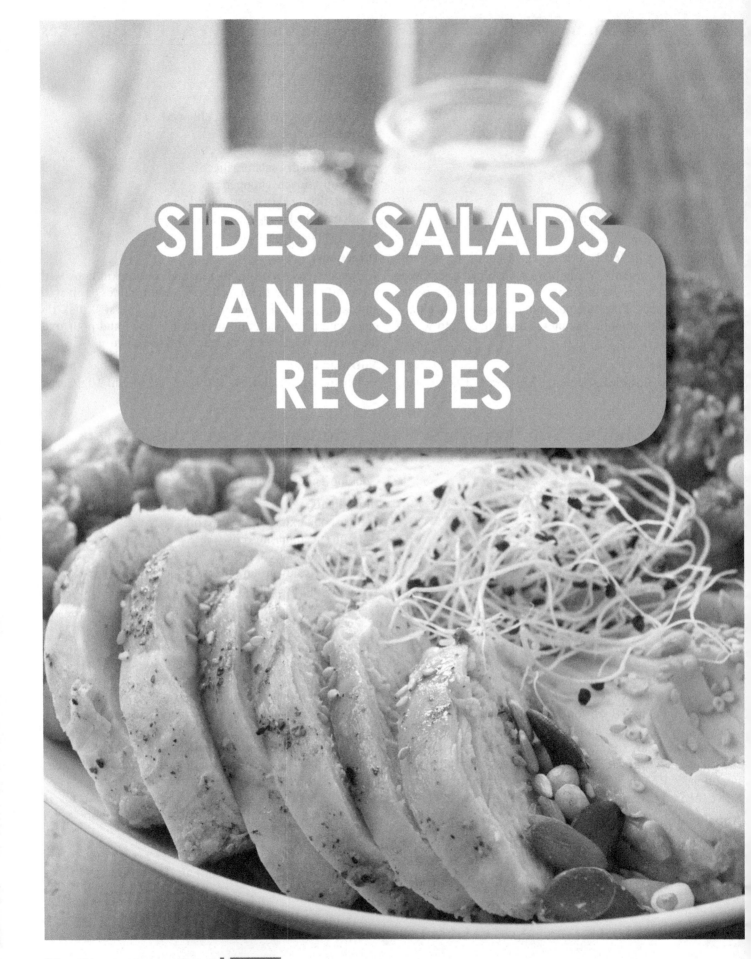

SIDES , SALADS, AND SOUPS RECIPES

Sides , Salads, And Soups Recipes

Vegetable Feta Bake

Servings:6
Cooking Time:30 Minutes

Ingredients:
- 2 tbsp olive oil
- 1 medium onion, sliced
- 1 green bell pepper, chopped
- 1 red bell pepper, chopped
- ½ lb feta cheese slice
- 1 tsp dried oregano
- Black pepper to taste
- ½ lb cherry tomatoes, halved

Directions:
1. Preheat oven to 350 F. Warm the olive oil in a pan over medium heat. Add and sauté the onion and bell peppers for 6-8 minutes until soft. Place the feta in a small greased baking dish and top with sautéed vegetables. Top with oregano and black pepper. Arrange the cherry tomatoes around the cheese. Cover with foil and bake for 13-15 minutes.

Nutrition Info:
- Per Serving: Calories: 153;Fat: 13g;Protein: 6g;Carbs: 5g.

Classic Tzatziki

Servings:6
Cooking Time:5 Minutes

Ingredients:
- 2 Persian cucumbers, chopped
- 3 cups Greek yogurt
- 2 garlic cloves, minced
- Salt to taste
- 1 tsp dried dill
- 1 tbsp olive oil
- ½ lemon, juiced

Directions:
1. Using a paper towel, squeeze out the excess liquid from the cucumbers. Place them into a bowl and pour in the yogurt, garlic, salt, and lemon. Stir in the oil, and top the dill. Mix well and serve at room temperature or chilled.

Nutrition Info:
- Per Serving: Calories: 127;Fat: 6g;Protein: 10.9g;Carbs: 7.1g.

Leek & Shrimp Soup

Servings:6
Cooking Time:40 Minutes

Ingredients:
- 1 lb shrimp, peeled and deveined
- 3 tbsp olive oil
- 1 celery stalk, chopped
- 1 leek, sliced
- 1 fennel bulb, chopped
- 2 garlic cloves, minced
- Salt and black pepper to taste
- 1 tbsp coriander seeds
- 6 cups vegetable broth
- 2 tbsp buttermilk
- 1 lemon, juiced

Directions:
1. Warm the oil in a large pot oven over medium heat. Add the celery, leek, and fennel, and cook for about 5 minutes until tender. Add the garlic and season with salt and pepper. Add the coriander seeds and stir. Pour in the broth, bring to a boil, and then reduce to a simmer and cook for 20 more minutes. Add the shrimp to the soup and cook until just pink, about 3 minutes. Stir in buttermilk and lemon juice. Serve.

Nutrition Info:
- Per Serving: Calories: 286;Fat: 9g;Protein: 17g;Carbs: 34g.

Three-bean Salad

Servings:4
Cooking Time:20 Minutes

Ingredients:
- 2 tbsp olive oil
- ½ cup white beans, cooked
- ½ cup fava beans, cooked
- ½ cup lima beans, cooked
- 1 red bell pepper, diced
- 2 tbsp parsley, chopped
- 1 tsp ground cumin
- 1 celery stalk, finely chopped
- 1 lemon, juiced
- Salt and black pepper to taste

Directions:
1. Place the olive oil, beans, bell pepper, parsley, cumin,

lemon juice, celery, salt, and pepper in a large bowl and mix well. Season to taste. Allow to sit for 5 minutes, so the flavors can come together before serving.

Nutrition Info:
- Per Serving: Calories: 223;Fat: 7.7g;Protein: 11g;Carbs: 30g.

Bell Pepper, Tomato & Egg Salad

Servings:4
Cooking Time:15 Min + Chilling Time

Ingredients:
- 4 tbsp olive oil
- 2 hard-boiled eggs, chopped
- 2 cups Greek yogurt
- 1 cup tomatoes, chopped
- 2 mixed bell peppers, sliced
- 1 yellow onion, thinly sliced
- ½ tsp fresh garlic, minced
- 10 Kalamata olives, sliced
- 3 sun-dried tomatoes, chopped
- 1 tbsp fresh lemon juice
- 1 tsp dill, chopped
- 2 tbsp fresh parsley, chopped
- Salt and black pepper to taste

Directions:
1. In a bowl, combine the bell peppers, onion, garlic, Kalamata olives, chopped tomatoes, and sun-dried tomatoes. Stir in the chopped eggs. For the dressing, combine the lemon juice, olive oil, Greek yogurt, dill, salt, and black pepper in a bowl. Pour over the salad and transfer to the fridge to chill. Serve garnished with olives and parsley.

Nutrition Info:
- Per Serving: Calories: 279;Fat: 19g;Protein: 14g;Carbs: 14g.

Mushroom & Parmesan Risotto

Servings:4
Cooking Time:25 Minutes

Ingredients:
- 1 ½ cups mixed mushrooms, sliced
- 3 tbsp olive oil
- 1 shallot, chopped
- 1 cup Arborio rice
- 4 cups vegetable stock
- 2 tbsp dry white wine
- 1 cup grated Parmesan cheese
- 2 tbsp butter
- 2 tbsp fresh parsley, chopped

Directions:
1. Pour the vegetable stock into a small saucepan over low heat and bring to a simmer; then turn the heat off.
2. Warm the olive oil in a large saucepan over medium heat. Sauté the mushrooms and shallot for 6 minutes until tender. Stir in rice for 3 minutes until opaque. Pour in the wine and stir. Gradually add the hot stock to the rice mixture, about 1 ladleful at a time, stirring until the liquid is absorbed. Remove the saucepan from the heat, stir in butter and 3 tbsp of Parmesan cheese. Cover and leave to rest for 5 minutes. Scatter the remaining cheese and parsley over the risotto and serve in bowls.

Nutrition Info:
- Per Serving: Calories: 354;Fat: 29g;Protein: 11g;Carbs: 22g.

Restaurant-style Zuppa Di Fagioli

Servings:4
Cooking Time:10 Minutes

Ingredients:
- 2 tbsp Pecorino cheese, grated
- 2 tbsp olive oil
- 1 carrot, peeled and diced
- 1 onion, chopped
- 2 cloves garlic, chopped
- 4 cups chicken broth
- ½ cup white beans, soaked
- 1 tsp dried thyme
- Salt and black pepper to taste
- 4 whole-wheat bread slices

Directions:
1. Warm the olive oil in a large stockpot over medium heat. Add the carrot and onion and sauté until the onion is translucent. Stir-fry the garlic for 1 more minute. Pour in the broth, beans, salt, and pepper, and cover. Bring to a boil and simmer for 2 hours or until the beans are tender. Adjust the taste and top with Pecorino cheese. Serve with toasted whole-wheat bread.

Nutrition Info:
- Per Serving: Calories: 186;Fat: 3g;Protein: 6g;Carbs: 24g.

Mediterranean Tomato Hummus Soup

Servings:2
Cooking Time: 10 Minutes

Ingredients:
- 1 can crushed tomatoes with basil
- 2 cups low-sodium chicken stock
- 1 cup roasted red pepper hummus
- Salt, to taste
- ¼ cup thinly sliced fresh basil leaves, for garnish (optional)

Directions:

1. Combine the canned tomatoes, hummus, and chicken stock in a blender and blend until smooth. Pour the mixture into a saucepan and bring it to a boil. Season with salt to taste.

2. Serve garnished with the fresh basil, if desired.

Nutrition Info:
• Per Serving: Calories: 147;Fat: 6.2g;Protein: 5.2g;Carbs: 20.1g.

Mushroom & Bell Pepper Salad

Servings:4
Cooking Time:15 Minutes

Ingredients:
• 2 tbsp olive oil
• ½ lb mushrooms, sliced
• 3 garlic cloves, minced
• Salt and black pepper to taste
• 1 tomato, diced
• 1 red bell pepper, sliced
• 3 tbsp lime juice
• ½ cup chicken stock
• 2 tbsp cilantro, chopped

Directions:

1. Warm the olive oil in a skillet over medium heat and sauté mushrooms for 4 minutes. Stir in garlic, salt, pepper, tomato, bell pepper, lime juice, and chicken stock and sauté for another 4 minutes. Top with cilantro and serve right away.

Nutrition Info:
• Per Serving: Calories: 89;Fat: 7.4g;Protein: 2.5g;Carbs: 5.6g.

Arugula, Watermelon, And Feta Salad

Servings:2
Cooking Time: 0 Minutes

Ingredients:
• 3 cups packed arugula
• 2½ cups watermelon, cut into bite-size cubes
• 2 ounces feta cheese, crumbled
• 2 tablespoons balsamic glaze

Directions:

1. Divide the arugula between two plates.

2. Divide the watermelon cubes between the beds of arugula.

3. Scatter half of the feta cheese over each salad.

4. Drizzle about 1 tablespoon of the glaze (or more if desired) over each salad. Serve immediately.

Nutrition Info:
• Per Serving: Calories: 157;Fat: 6.9g;Protein: 6.1g;Carbs: 22.0g.

Radish & Pecorino Salad

Servings:6
Cooking Time:15 Minutes

Ingredients:
• 6 tbsp grated Pecorino Romano cheese
• ¼ cup extra-virgin olive oil
• 6 cups kale, chopped
• 2 tbsp lemon juice
• Salt to taste
• 2 cups arugula
• ⅓ cup shelled pistachios
• 20 radishes, sliced

Directions:

1. In a salad bowl, whisk the olive oil, lemon juice, and salt. Add the kale and gently massage the leaves with your hands for about 15 seconds until all are thoroughly coated. Let the kale sit for 5 minutes. Add in the arugula, radishes, and pistachios and toss. Sprinkle with Pecorino and serve.

Nutrition Info:
• Per Serving: Calories: 105;Fat: 9.2g;Protein: 4g;Carbs: 3.8g.

Carrot & Rice Salad

Servings:4
Cooking Time:10 Minutes

Ingredients:
• 2 tbsp olive oil
• 1 head Iceberg lettuce, torn
• 2 carrots, grated
• 1 cup brown rice, cooked
• 1 red onion, sliced
• ½ cup mint, chopped
• 1 lime, juiced
• ½ cup corn
• Salt and black pepper to taste

Directions:

1. Mix rice, olive oil, onion, lettuce, carrot, mint, lime juice, corn, salt, and pepper in a bowl. Serve right away.

Nutrition Info:
• Per Serving: Calories: 160;Fat: 7g;Protein: 7g;Carbs: 10g.

Feta & Olive Salad

Servings:4
Cooking Time:10 Minutes

Ingredients:
- ½ cup extra-virgin olive oil
- 1 head iceberg lettuce, torn
- 2 tomatoes, sliced
- 1 cucumber, sliced
- 1 red onion, thinly sliced
- ¼ cup lemon juice
- Salt to taste
- 1 clove garlic, minced
- 1 cup Kalamata olives, pitted
- 6 oz feta cheese, crumbled
- 2 tbsp dill, chopped

Directions:
1. Place the lettuce in a large salad bowl. Add the tomatoes, cucumber, onion, and dill. In another small bowl, whisk together the olive oil, lemon juice, salt, and garlic. Pour the dressing over the salad and gently toss to evenly coat. Sprinkle the salad with the Kalamata olives and feta cheese. Serve and enjoy!

Nutrition Info:
- Per Serving: Calories: 539;Fat: 50.2g;Protein: 9g;Carbs: 18g.

Lemon-tahini Hummus

Servings:6
Cooking Time: 0 Minutes

Ingredients:
- 1 can chickpeas, drained and rinsed
- 4 tablespoons extra-virgin olive oil, divided
- 4 to 5 tablespoons tahini (sesame seed paste)
- 2 lemons, juiced
- 1 lemon, zested, divided
- 1 tablespoon minced garlic
- Pinch salt

Directions:
1. In a food processor, combine the chickpeas, 2 tablespoons of olive oil, tahini, lemon juice, half of the lemon zest, and garlic and pulse for up to 1 minute, scraping down the sides of the food processor bowl as necessary.
2. Taste and add salt as needed. Feel free to add 1 teaspoon of water at a time to thin the hummus to a better consistency.
3. Transfer the hummus to a serving bowl. Serve drizzled with the remaining 2 tablespoons of olive oil and remaining half of the lemon zest.

Nutrition Info:
- Per Serving: Calories: 216;Fat: 15.0g;Protein: 5.0g;-

Carbs: 17.0g.

Parsley Garden Vegetable Soup

Servings:4
Cooking Time:25 Minutes

Ingredients:
- ¼ head green cabbage, shredded
- 2 tbsp olive oil
- 1 cup leeks, chopped
- 2 garlic cloves, minced
- 8 cups vegetable stock
- 1 carrot, diced
- 1 potato, diced
- 1 celery stalk, diced
- 1 cup mushrooms
- 1 cup broccoli florets
- 1 cup cauliflower florets
- ½ red bell pepper, diced
- ½ cup green beans
- Salt and black pepper to taste
- 2 tbsp fresh parsley, chopped

Directions:
1. Heat oil on Sauté in your Instant Pot. Add in garlic and leeks and cook for 6 minutes until slightly browned. Add in stock, carrot, celery, broccoli, bell pepper, green beans, salt, cabbage, cauliflower, mushrooms, potato, and pepper. Seal lid and cook on High Pressure for 6 minutes. Release pressure naturally for about 10 minutes. Stir in parsley and serve.

Nutrition Info:
- Per Serving: Calories: 218;Fat: 7g;Protein: 5g;Carbs: 36g.

Greek Salad

Servings:4
Cooking Time:10 Minutes

Ingredients:
- 2 tbsp extra-virgin olive oil
- 2 tomatoes, chopped
- ½ cup grated feta cheese
- 1 green bell pepper, chopped
- 10 Kalamata olives, chopped
- 1 red onion, thinly sliced
- 1 cucumber, chopped
- 2 tbsp apple cider vinegar
- 1 tbsp dried oregano
- Salt and black pepper to taste
- 2 tbsp fresh parsley, chopped

Directions:
1. In a salad bowl, combine bell pepper, red onion, tomatoes, cucumber, and olives. Mix the olive oil, apple cider

vinegar, oregano, salt, and pepper in another bowl. Pour the dressing over the salad and toss to combine. Top with the feta cheese and sprinkle with parsley to serve.

Nutrition Info:
- Per Serving: Calories: 172;Fat: 13g;Protein: 4.4g;Carbs: 12g.

Chickpea & Broccoli Salad

Servings:6
Cooking Time:10 Minutes

Ingredients:
- ¼ cup extra-virgin olive oil
- 10 oz broccoli florets, steamed
- 2 cans chickpeas
- 15 cherry tomatoes, halved
- ½ red onion, finely chopped
- 2 lemons, juiced and zested
- 2 garlic cloves, minced
- 2 tsp dried oregano
- Salt and black pepper to taste

Directions:
1. Mix the chickpeas, red onion, cherry tomatoes, and broccoli in a bowl. Combine the olive oil, lemon juice, lemon zest, oregano, garlic, salt, and pepper in another bowl. Pour over the salad and toss to combine. Serve immediately.

Nutrition Info:
- Per Serving: Calories: 569;Fat: 16g;Protein: 26g;Carbs: 84g.

Zucchini & Green Bean Soup

Servings:4
Cooking Time:30 Minutes

Ingredients:
- 1 ¼ lb green beans, cut into bite-sized chunks
- 2 tbsp olive oil
- 1 onion, chopped
- 1 celery with leaves, chopped
- 1 carrot, chopped
- 2 garlic cloves, minced
- 1 zucchini, chopped
- 5 cups vegetable broth
- 2 tomatoes, chopped
- Salt and black pepper to taste
- ½ tsp cayenne pepper
- 1 tsp oregano
- ½ tsp dried dill
- ½ cup black olives, sliced

Directions:
1. Warm the olive in a pot over medium heat. Sauté the onion, celery, and carrot for about 4 minutes or until the veg-

etables are just tender. Add in the garlic and zucchini and continue to sauté for 1 minute or until aromatic. Pour in the broth, green beans, tomatoes, salt, black pepper, cayenne pepper, oregano, and dried dill; bring to a boil. Reduce the heat to a simmer and let it cook for about 15 minutes. Serve in individual bowls with sliced olives.

Nutrition Info:
- Per Serving: Calories: 315;Fat: 24g;Protein: 16g;Carbs: 14g.

Mushroom & Spinach Orzo Soup

Servings:4
Cooking Time:20 Minutes

Ingredients:
- 2 tbsp butter
- 3 cups spinach
- ½ cup orzo
- 4 cups chicken broth
- 1 cup feta cheese, crumbled
- Salt and black pepper to taste
- ½ tsp dried oregano
- 1 onion, chopped
- 2 garlic cloves, minced
- 1 cup mushrooms, sliced

Directions:
1. Melt butter in a pot over medium heat and sauté onion, garlic, and mushrooms for 5 minutes until tender. Add in chicken broth, orzo, salt, pepper, and oregano. Bring to a boil and reduce the heat to a low. Continue simmering for 10 minutes, partially covered. Stir in spinach and continue to cook until the spinach wilts, about 3-4 minutes. Ladle into individual bowls and serve garnished with feta cheese.

Nutrition Info:
- Per Serving: Calories: 370;Fat: 11g;Protein: 23g;Carbs: 44g.

Garlic Wilted Greens

Servings:2
Cooking Time: 5 Minutes

Ingredients:
- 1 tablespoon olive oil
- 2 garlic cloves, minced
- 3 cups sliced greens (spinach, chard, beet greens, dandelion greens, or a combination)
- Pinch salt
- Pinch red pepper flakes (or more to taste)

Directions:
1. Heat the olive oil in a skillet over medium-high heat.
2. Add garlic and sauté for 30 seconds, or just until fragrant.

3. Add the greens, salt, and pepper flakes and stir to combine. Let the greens wilt, but do not overcook.
4. Remove from the skillet and serve on a plate.

Nutrition Info:
• Per Serving: Calories: 93;Fat: 6.8g;Protein: 1.2g;Carbs: 7.3g.

Barley, Parsley, And Pea Salad

Servings:4
Cooking Time: 10 Minutes

Ingredients:
• 2 cups water
• 1 cup quick-cooking barley
• 1 small bunch flat-leaf parsley, chopped
• 2 cups sugar snap pea pods
• Juice of 1 lemon
• ½ small red onion, diced
• 2 tablespoons extra-virgin olive oil
• Sea salt and freshly ground pepper, to taste

Directions:
1. Pour the water in a saucepan. Bring to a boil. Add the barley to the saucepan, then put the lid on.
2. Reduce the heat to low. Simmer the barley for 10 minutes or until the liquid is absorbed, then let sit for 5 minutes.
3. Open the lid, then transfer the barley in a colander and rinse under cold running water.
4. Pour the barley in a large salad bowl and add the remaining ingredients. Toss to combine well.
5. Serve immediately.

Nutrition Info:
• Per Serving: Calories: 152;Fat: 7.4g;Protein: 3.7g;Carbs: 19.3g.

Mackerel & Radish Salad

Servings:4
Cooking Time:5 Minutes

Ingredients:
• 3 tbsp olive oil
• 4 oz smoked mackerel, flaked
• 10 radishes, sliced
• 5 oz baby arugula
• 1 cup corn
• 2 tbsp lemon juice
• Sea salt to taste
• 2 tbsp fresh parsley, chopped

Directions:
1. Place the arugula on a serving plate. Top with corn, mackerel, and radishes.Mix olive oil, lemon juice, and salt in a bowl and pour the dressing over the salad. Top with parsley.

Nutrition Info:
• Per Serving: Calories: 300;Fat: 19g;Protein: 19g;Carbs: 23g.

Chicken And Pastina Soup

Servings:6
Cooking Time: 20 Minutes

Ingredients:
• 1 tablespoon extra-virgin olive oil
• 2 garlic cloves, minced
• 3 cups packed chopped kale, center ribs removed
• 1 cup minced carrots
• 8 cups no-salt-added chicken or vegetable broth
• ¼ teaspoon kosher or sea salt
• ¼ teaspoon freshly ground black pepper
• ¾ cup uncooked acini de pepe or pastina pasta
• 2 cups shredded cooked chicken
• 3 tablespoons grated Parmesan cheese

Directions:
1. In a large stockpot over medium heat, heat the oil. Add the garlic and cook for 30 seconds, stirring frequently. Add the kale and carrots and cook for 5 minutes, stirring occasionally.
2. Add the broth, salt, and pepper, and turn the heat to high. Bring the broth to a boil, and add the pasta. Reduce the heat to medium and cook for 10 minutes, or until the pasta is cooked through, stirring every few minutes so the pasta doesn't stick to the bottom. Add the chicken, and cook for another 2 minutes to warm through.
3. Ladle the soup into six bowls. Top each with ½ tablespoon of cheese and serve.

Nutrition Info:
• Per Serving: Calories: 275;Fat: 19.0g;Protein: 16.0g;-Carbs: 11.0g.

Roasted Red Pepper & Olive Spread

Servings:6
Cooking Time:10 Minutes

Ingredients:
• ¼ tsp dried thyme
• 1 tbsp capers
• ½ cup pitted green olives
• 1 roasted red pepper, chopped
• 1 tsp balsamic vinegar
• 2⁄3 cup soft bread crumbs
• 2 cloves garlic, minced
• ½ tsp red pepper flakes
• 1⁄3 cup extra-virgin olive oil

Directions:
1. Place all the ingredients, except for the olive oil, in a food processor and blend until chunky. With the machine

running, slowly pour in the olive oil until it is well combined. Refrigerate or serve at room temperature.

Nutrition Info:
- Per Serving: Calories: 467;Fat: 38g;Protein: 5g;Carbs: 27g.

Home-style Harissa Paste

Servings:4
Cooking Time:10 Minutes

Ingredients:
- 1 tbsp ground dried Aleppo pepper
- 1 tbsp lemon juice
- 2 tbsp tomato paste
- 6 tbsp extra-virgin olive oil
- 6 garlic cloves, minced
- 2 tbsp paprika
- 1 tbsp ground coriander
- 1 tsp ground cumin
- ¾ tsp caraway seeds
- ½ tsp salt

Directions:
1. Microwave the oil, garlic, paprika, coriander, Aleppo pepper, cumin, caraway seeds, and salt for about 1 minute until bubbling and very fragrant, stirring halfway through microwaving. Let cool at room temperature. Store in an airtight container in the refrigerator for up to 2-3 days.

Nutrition Info:
- Per Serving: Calories: 162;Fat: 8.4g;Protein: 4.7g;Carbs: 9g.

Traditional Dukkah Spice

Servings:6
Cooking Time:50 Minutes

Ingredients:
- ⅓ cup black sesame seeds, toasted
- 1 tsp olive oil
- 1 can chickpeas
- ½ cup almonds, toasted
- 2 tbsp coriander seeds
- 1 tbsp cumin seeds, toasted
- 2 tsp fennel seeds, toasted
- Salt and black pepper to taste

Directions:
1. Preheat oven to 400 F. Spread the chickpeas in a single layer on a baking sheet and drizzle with olive oil. Roast for 40-45 minutes until browned and crisp, stirring every 5-10 minutes. Remove and let cool completely.
2. Blend the remaining ingredients in your food processor and remove to a bowl. Pour the cooled chickpeas into the food processor and pulse until coarsely ground. Mix them

with the almonds and seeds until well combined. Store the spices in an airtight container at room temperature for up to 1 month.

Nutrition Info:
- Per Serving: Calories: 198;Fat: 3.0g;Protein: 2.1g;Carbs: 5g.

Harissa Chicken Wings

Servings:4
Cooking Time:45 Min + Marinating Time

Ingredients:
- ½ tsp harissa seasoning
- 4 garlic cloves, minced
- 1 shallot, grated
- 1 tbsp lemon zest
- 1 tbsp lemon juice
- ¼ tsp ground cinnamon
- ¼ tsp smoked paprika
- ½ tsp ground allspice
- Salt and black pepper to taste
- 2 tbsp fresh thyme, chopped
- ¼ cup extra-virgin olive oil
- 2 lb chicken wings

Directions:
1. Combine all ingredients, except for the chicken wings, in a bowl. Add the chicken and toss to coat. Refrigerate for 2 hours. Preheat oven to 425 F. Remove wings from the refrigerator and discard the excess marinade from them. Arrange the wings on a parchment-lined baking sheet. Bake for 30-35 minutes, flipping once until crispy and brown.

Nutrition Info:
- Per Serving: Calories: 417;Fat: 22g;Protein: 50g;Carbs: 3g.

Roasted Broccoli And Tomato Panzanella

Servings:4
Cooking Time: 20 Minutes

Ingredients:
- 1 pound broccoli, trimmed, cut into 1-inch florets and ½-inch stem slices
- 2 tablespoons extra-virgin olive oil, divided
- 1½ cups cherry tomatoes
- 1½ teaspoons honey, divided
- 3 cups cubed whole-grain crusty bread
- 1 tablespoon balsamic vinegar
- ¼ teaspoon kosher salt
- ½ teaspoon freshly ground black pepper
- ¼ cup grated Parmesan cheese, for serving (optional)
- ¼ cup chopped fresh oregano leaves, for serving

(optional)

Directions:

1. Preheat the oven to 450ºF.

2. Toss the broccoli with 1 tablespoon of olive oil in a large bowl to coat well.

3. Arrange the broccoli on a baking sheet, then add the tomatoes to the same bowl and toss with the remaining olive oil. Add 1 teaspoon of honey and toss again to coat well. Transfer the tomatoes on the baking sheet beside the broccoli.

4. Place the baking sheet in the preheated oven and roast for 15 minutes, then add the bread cubes and flip the vegetables. Roast for an additional 3 minutes or until the broccoli is lightly charred and the bread cubes are golden brown.

5. Meanwhile, combine the remaining ingredients, except for the Parmesan and oregano, in a small bowl. Stir to mix well.

6. Transfer the roasted vegetables and bread cubes to the large salad bowl, then dress them and spread with Parmesan and oregano leaves. Toss and serve immediately.

Nutrition Info:

• Per Serving: Calories: 162;Fat: 6.8g;Protein: 8.2g;Carbs: 18.9g.

Paella Soup

Servings:6
Cooking Time: 24 Minutes

Ingredients:

• 2 tablespoons extra-virgin olive oil
• 1 cup chopped onion
• 1½ cups coarsely chopped green bell pepper
• 1½ cups coarsely chopped red bell pepper
• 2 garlic cloves, chopped
• 1 teaspoon ground turmeric
• 1 teaspoon dried thyme
• 2 teaspoons smoked paprika
• 2½ cups uncooked instant brown rice
• 2 cups low-sodium or no-salt-added chicken broth
• 2½ cups water
• 1 cup frozen green peas, thawed
• 1 can low-sodium or no-salt-added crushed tomatoes
• 1 pound fresh raw medium shrimp, shells and tails removed

Directions:

1. In a large stockpot over medium-high heat, heat the oil. Add the onion, bell peppers, and garlic. Cook for 8 minutes, stirring occasionally. Add the turmeric, thyme, and smoked paprika, and cook for 2 minutes more, stirring often. Stir in the rice, broth, and water. Bring to a boil over high heat. Cover, reduce the heat to medium-low, and cook for 10 minutes.

2. Stir the peas, tomatoes, and shrimp into the soup. Cook for 4 minutes, until the shrimp is cooked, turning from gray to pink and white. The soup will be very thick, almost like stew, when ready to serve.

3. Ladle the soup into bowls and serve hot.

Nutrition Info:

• Per Serving: Calories: 431;Fat: 5.7g;Protein: 26.0g;-Carbs: 69.1g.

Rich Chicken And Small Pasta Broth

Servings:6
Cooking Time: 4 Hours

Ingredients:

• 6 boneless, skinless chicken thighs
• 4 stalks celery, cut into ½-inch pieces
• 4 carrots, cut into 1-inch pieces
• 1 medium yellow onion, halved
• 2 garlic cloves, minced
• 2 bay leaves
• Sea salt and freshly ground black pepper, to taste
• 6 cups low-sodium chicken stock
• ½ cup stelline pasta
• ¼ cup chopped fresh flat-leaf parsley

Directions:

1. Combine the chicken thighs, celery, carrots, onion, and garlic in the slow cooker. Spread with bay leaves and sprinkle with salt and pepper. Toss to mix well.

2. Pour in the chicken stock. Put the lid on and cook on high for 4 hours or until the internal temperature of chicken reaches at least 165ºF.

3. In the last 20 minutes of the cooking, remove the chicken from the slow cooker and transfer to a bowl to cool until ready to reserve.

4. Discard the bay leaves and add the pasta to the slow cooker. Put the lid on and cook for 15 minutes or until al dente.

5. Meanwhile, slice the chicken, then put the chicken and parsley in the slow cooker and cook for 5 minutes or until well combined.

6. Pour the soup in a large bowl and serve immediately.

Nutrition Info:

• Per Serving: Calories: 285;Fat: 10.8g;Protein: 27.4g;-Carbs: 18.8g.

White Bean Soup With Farro

Servings:6
Cooking Time:2 Hours 10 Minutes

Ingredients:
- 1 can diced tomatoes, with juice
- 2 tbsp olive oil
- 1 onion, diced
- 1 celery stalk, diced
- 2 garlic cloves, minced
- 6 cups chicken broth
- 1 cup white beans, soaked
- 1 cup farro
- ½ tsp rosemary
- Salt and black pepper to taste

Directions:
1. Warm the olive oil in a large stockpot over medium heat. Sauté the onion, celery, and garlic cloves just until tender. Add the broth, beans, tomatoes, farro, and seasonings, and bring to a simmer. Cover and cook for 2 hours or until the beans and farro are tender. Season with salt and pepper.

Nutrition Info:
- Per Serving: Calories: 595;Fat: 21g;Protein: 60g;Carbs: 38g.

Paprika Bean Soup

Servings:4
Cooking Time:50 Minutes

Ingredients:
- 2 tbsp olive oil
- 6 cups veggie stock
- 1 cup celery, chopped
- 1 cup carrots, chopped
- 1 yellow onion, chopped
- 2 garlic cloves, minced
- ½ cup navy beans, soaked
- 2 tbsp chopped parsley
- ½ tsp paprika
- 1 tsp thyme
- Salt and black pepper to taste

Directions:
1. Warm olive oil in a saucepan and sauté onion, garlic, carrots, and celery for 5 minutes, stirring occasionally. Stir in paprika, thyme, salt, and pepper for 1 minute. Pour in broth and navy beans. Bring to a boil, then reduce the heat and simmer for 40 minutes. Sprinkle with parsley and serve.

Nutrition Info:
- Per Serving: Calories: 270;Fat: 18g;Protein: 12g;Carbs: 24g.

Greek Chicken, Tomato, And Olive Salad

Servings:2
Cooking Time: 0 Minutes

Ingredients:
- Salad:
- 2 grilled boneless, skinless chicken breasts, sliced
- 10 cherry tomatoes, halved
- 8 pitted Kalamata olives, halved
- ½ cup thinly sliced red onion
- Dressing:
- ¼ cup balsamic vinegar
- 1 teaspoon freshly squeezed lemon juice
- ¼ teaspoon sea salt
- ¼ teaspoon freshly ground black pepper
- 2 teaspoons extra-virgin olive oil
- For Serving:
- 2 cups roughly chopped romaine lettuce
- ½ cup crumbled feta cheese

Directions:
1. Combine the ingredients for the salad in a large bowl. Toss to combine well.
2. Combine the ingredients for the dressing in a small bowl. Stir to mix well.
3. Pour the dressing the bowl of salad, then toss to coat well. Wrap the bowl in plastic and refrigerate for at least 2 hours.
4. Remove the bowl from the refrigerator. Spread the lettuce on a large plate, then top with marinated salad. Scatter the salad with feta cheese and serve immediately.

Nutrition Info:
- Per Serving: Calories: 328;Fat: 16.9g;Protein: 27.6g;Carbs: 15.9g.

Yogurt Cucumber Salad

Servings:4
Cooking Time:10 Min + Chilling Time

Ingredients:
- 1 tbsp olive oil
- 2 tbsp walnuts, ground
- 1 cup Greek yogurt
- 2 garlic cloves, minced
- Salt and white pepper to taste
- 1 tbsp wine vinegar
- 1 tbsp dill, chopped
- 3 medium cucumbers, sliced
- 1 tbsp chives, chopped

Directions:
1. Combine cucumbers, walnuts, garlic, salt, pepper, vinegar, yogurt, dill, olive oil, and chives in a bowl. Let sit in the fridge for 1 hour. Serve.

Nutrition Info:
- Per Serving: Calories: 220;Fat: 13g;Protein: 4g;Carbs: 9g.

Three-bean Salad With Black Olives

Servings:6
Cooking Time:15 Minutes

Ingredients:
- 1 lb green beans, trimmed
- 1 red onion, thinly sliced
- 2 tbsp marjoram, chopped
- ¼ cup black olives, chopped
- ½ cup canned cannellini beans
- ½ cup canned chickpeas
- 2 tbsp extra-virgin olive oil
- ½ cup balsamic vinegar
- ½ tsp dried oregano
- Salt and black pepper to taste

Directions:
1. Steam the green beans for about 2 minutes or until just tender. Drain and place them in an ice-water bath. Drain thoroughly and pat them dry with paper towels. Put them in a large bowl and toss with the remaining ingredients. Serve.

Nutrition Info:
- Per Serving: Calories: 187;Fat: 6g;Protein: 7g;Carbs: 27g.

Balsamic Brussels Sprouts And Delicata Squash

Servings:2
Cooking Time: 30 Minutes

Ingredients:
- ½ pound Brussels sprouts, ends trimmed and outer leaves removed
- 1 medium delicata squash, halved lengthwise, seeded, and cut into 1-inch pieces
- 1 cup fresh cranberries
- 2 teaspoons olive oil
- Salt and freshly ground black pepper, to taste
- ½ cup balsamic vinegar
- 2 tablespoons roasted pumpkin seeds
- 2 tablespoons fresh pomegranate arils (seeds)

Directions:
1. Preheat oven to 400ºF. Line a sheet pan with parchment paper.
2. Combine the Brussels sprouts, squash, and cranberries in a large bowl. Drizzle with olive oil, and season lightly with salt and pepper. Toss well to coat and arrange in a single layer on the sheet pan.
3. Roast in the preheated oven for 30 minutes, turning vegetables halfway through, or until Brussels sprouts turn brown and crisp in spots.
4. Meanwhile, make the balsamic glaze by simmering the vinegar for 10 to 12 minutes, or until mixture has reduced to about ¼ cup and turns a syrupy consistency.
5. Remove the vegetables from the oven, drizzle with balsamic syrup, and sprinkle with pumpkin seeds and pomegranate arils before serving.

Nutrition Info:
- Per Serving: Calories: 203;Fat: 6.8g;Protein: 6.2g;Carbs: 22.0g.

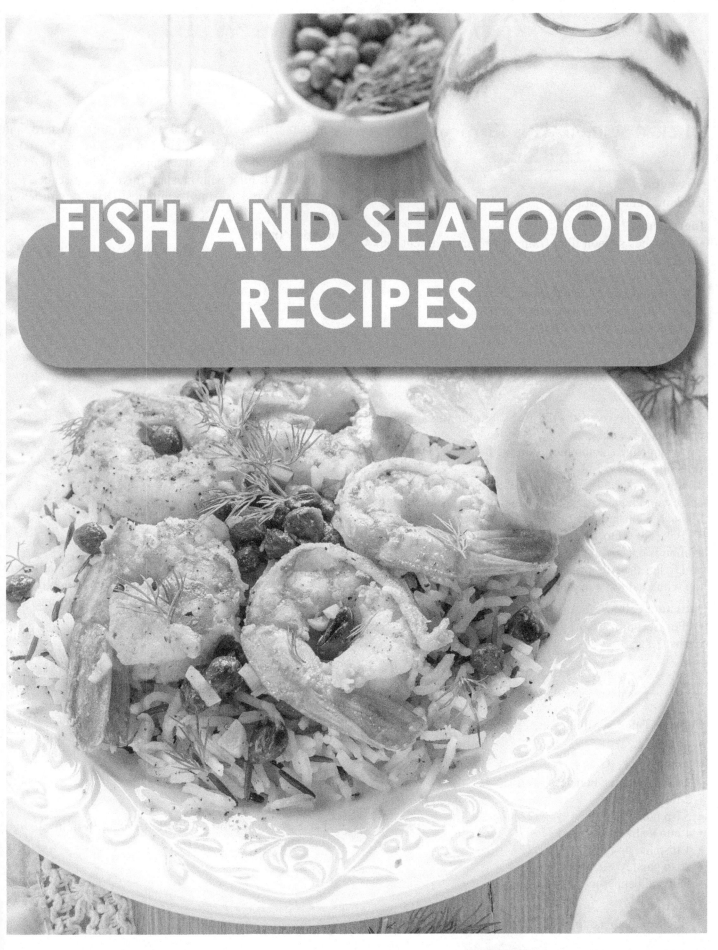

FISH AND SEAFOOD RECIPES

Fish And Seafood Recipes

Baked Salmon With Tarragon Mustard Sauce

Servings:4
Cooking Time: 12 Minutes

Ingredients:
- 1¼ pounds salmon fillet (skin on or removed), cut into 4 equal pieces
- ¼ cup Dijon mustard
- ¼ cup avocado oil mayonnaise
- Zest and juice of ½ lemon
- 2 tablespoons chopped fresh tarragon
- ½ teaspoon salt
- ¼ teaspoon freshly ground black pepper
- 4 tablespoons extra-virgin olive oil, for serving

Directions:
1. Preheat the oven to 425°F. Line a baking sheet with parchment paper.
2. Arrange the salmon pieces on the prepared baking sheet, skin-side down.
3. Stir together the mustard, avocado oil mayonnaise, lemon zest and juice, tarragon, salt, and pepper in a small bowl. Spoon the mustard mixture over the salmon.
4. Bake for 10 to 12 minutes, or until the top is golden and salmon is opaque in the center.
5. Divide the salmon among four plates and drizzle each top with 1 tablespoon of olive oil before serving.

Nutrition Info:
- Per Serving: Calories: 386;Fat: 27.7g;Protein: 29.3g;-Carbs: 3.8g.

Walnut-crusted Salmon

Servings:4
Cooking Time:25 Minutes

Ingredients:
- 2 tbsp olive oil
- 4 salmon fillets, boneless
- 2 tbsp mustard
- 5 tsp honey
- 1 cup walnuts, chopped
- 1 tbsp lemon juice
- 2 tsp parsley, chopped
- Salt and pepper to the taste

Directions:
1. Preheat the oven to 380F. Line a baking tray with parchment paper. In a bowl, whisk the olive oil, mustard, and honey. In a separate bowl, combine walnuts and parsley. Sprinkle salmon with salt and pepper and place them on the tray. Rub each fillet with mustard mixture and scatter with walnut mixture; bake for 15 minutes. Drizzle with lemon juice.

Nutrition Info:
- Per Serving: Calories: 300;Fat: 16g;Protein: 17g;Carbs: 22g.

Mediterranean Grilled Sea Bass

Servings:6
Cooking Time: 20 Minutes

Ingredients:
- ¼ teaspoon onion powder
- ¼ teaspoon garlic powder
- ¼ teaspoon paprika
- Lemon pepper and sea salt to taste
- 2 pounds sea bass
- 3 tablespoons extra-virgin olive oil, divided
- 2 large cloves garlic, chopped
- 1 tablespoon chopped Italian flat leaf parsley

Directions:
1. Preheat the grill to high heat.
2. Place the onion powder, garlic powder, paprika, lemon pepper, and sea salt in a large bowl and stir to combine.
3. Dredge the fish in the spice mixture, turning until well coated.
4. Heat 2 tablespoon of olive oil in a small skillet. Add the garlic and parsley and cook for 1 to 2 minutes, stirring occasionally. Remove the skillet from the heat and set aside.
5. Brush the grill grates lightly with remaining 1 tablespoon olive oil.
6. Grill the fish for about 7 minutes. Flip the fish and drizzle with the garlic mixture and cook for an additional 7 minutes, or until the fish flakes when pressed lightly with a fork.
7. Serve hot.

Nutrition Info:
- Per Serving: Calories: 200;Fat: 10.3g;Protein: 26.9g;-Carbs: 0.6g.

Steamed Mussels With Spaghetti

Servings:4
Cooking Time:30 Minutes

Ingredients:
- 2 lb mussels, cleaned and beards removed
- 1 lb cooked spaghetti
- 3 tbsp butter
- 2 garlic cloves, minced
- 1 carrot, diced
- 1 onion, chopped
- 2 celery sticks, chopped
- 1 cup white wine
- 2 tbsp parsley, chopped
- ½ tsp red pepper flakes
- 1 lemon, juiced

Directions:
1. Melt butter in a saucepan over medium heat and sauté the garlic, carrot, onion, and celery for 4-5 minutes, stirring occasionally until softened. Add the mussels, white wine, and lemon juice, cover, and bring to a boil. Reduce the heat and steam the for 4-6 minutes. Discard any unopened mussels. Stir in spaghetti to coat. Sprinkle with parsley and red pepper flakes to serve.

Nutrition Info:
- Per Serving: Calories: 669;Fat: 16g;Protein: 41g;Carbs: 77g.

Andalusian Prawns With Capers

Servings:4
Cooking Time:25 Minutes

Ingredients:
- 1 lb prawns, peeled, deveined
- 2 tbsp olive oil
- 1 lemon, zested and juiced
- 2 tomatoes, chopped
- 1 cup spring onions, chopped
- 2 tbsp capers, chopped
- 2 tbsp dill, chopped
- Salt and black pepper to taste

Directions:
1. Warm the olive oil in a skillet over medium heat and cook onions and capers for 2-3 minutes. Stir in prawns, lemon zest, tomatoes, dill, salt, and pepper and cook for another 6 minutes. Serve drizzled with lemon juice.

Nutrition Info:
- Per Serving: Calories: 230;Fat: 14g;Protein: 6g;Carbs: 23g.

Prawns With Mushrooms

Servings:4
Cooking Time:25 Minutes

Ingredients:
- 1 lb tiger prawns, peeled and deveined
- 3 tbsp olive oil
- 2 green onions, sliced
- ½ lb white mushrooms, sliced
- 2 tbsp balsamic vinegar
- 2 tsp garlic, minced

Directions:
1. Warm the olive oil in a skillet over medium heat and cook green onions and garlic for 2 minutes. Stir in mushrooms and balsamic vinegar and cook for an additional 6 minutes. Put in prawns and cook for 4 minutes. Serve right away.

Nutrition Info:
- Per Serving: Calories: 260;Fat: 9g;Protein: 19g;Carbs: 13g.

Better-for-you Cod & Potatoes

Servings:4
Cooking Time:35 Minutes

Ingredients:
- 1 tbsp olive oil
- 2 cod fillets
- 1 tbsp basil, chopped
- Salt and black pepper to taste
- 2 potatoes, peeled and sliced
- 2 tsp turmeric powder
- 1 garlic clove, minced

Directions:
1. Preheat the oven to 360F. Spread the potatoes on a greased baking dish and season with salt and pepper. Bake for 10 minutes. Arrange the cod fillets on top of the potatoes, sprinkle with salt and pepper, and drizzle with some olive oil. Bake for 10-12 more minutes until the fish flakes easily.
2. Warm the remaining olive oil in a skillet over medium heat and sauté garlic for 1 minute. Stir in basil, salt, pepper, turmeric powder, and 3-4 tbsp of water; cook for another 2-3 minutes. Pour the sauce over the cod fillets and serve warm.

Nutrition Info:
- Per Serving: Calories: 300;Fat: 15g;Protein: 33g;Carbs: 28g.

Baked Halibut Steaks With Vegetables

Servings:4
Cooking Time: 20 Minutes

Ingredients:
- 2 teaspoon olive oil, divided
- 1 clove garlic, peeled and minced
- ½ cup minced onion
- 1 cup diced zucchini
- 2 cups diced fresh tomatoes
- 2 tablespoons chopped fresh basil
- ¼ teaspoon salt
- ¼ teaspoon ground black pepper
- 4 halibut steaks
- ⅓ cup crumbled feta cheese

Directions:
1. Preheat oven to 450ºF. Coat a shallow baking dish lightly with 1 teaspoon of olive oil.
2. In a medium saucepan, heat the remaining 1 teaspoon of olive oil.
3. Add the garlic, onion, and zucchini and mix well. Cook for 5 minutes, stirring occasionally, or until the zucchini is softened.
4. Remove the saucepan from the heat and stir in the tomatoes, basil, salt, and pepper.
5. Place the halibut steaks in the coated baking dish in a single layer. Spread the zucchini mixture evenly over the steaks. Scatter the top with feta cheese.
6. Bake in the preheated oven for about 15 minutes, or until the fish flakes when pressed lightly with a fork. Serve hot.

Nutrition Info:
- Per Serving: Calories: 258;Fat: 7.6g;Protein: 38.6g;-Carbs: 6.5g.

Creamy Halibut & Potato Soup

Servings:4
Cooking Time:25 Minutes

Ingredients:
- 3 gold potatoes, peeled and cubed
- 4 oz halibut fillets, boneless and cubed
- 2 tbsp olive oil
- 2 carrots, chopped
- 1 red onion, chopped
- Salt and white pepper to taste
- 4 cups fish stock
- ½ cup heavy cream
- 1 tbsp dill, chopped

Directions:
1. Warm the olive oil in a skillet over medium heat and cook the onion for 3 minutes. Put in potatoes, salt, pepper, carrots, and stock and bring to a boil. Cook for an addition-al 5-6 minutes. Stir in halibut, cream, and dill and simmer for another 5 minutes. Serve right away.

Nutrition Info:
- Per Serving: Calories: 215;Fat: 17g;Protein: 12g;Carbs: 7g.

Sole Piccata With Capers

Servings:4
Cooking Time: 17 Minutes

Ingredients:
- 1 teaspoon extra-virgin olive oil
- 4 sole fillets, patted dry
- 3 tablespoons almond butter
- 2 teaspoons minced garlic
- 2 tablespoons all-purpose flour
- 2 cups low-sodium chicken broth
- Juice and zest of ½ lemon
- 2 tablespoons capers

Directions:
1. Place a large skillet over medium-high heat and add the olive oil.
2. Sear the sole fillets until the fish flakes easily when tested with a fork, about 4 minutes on each side. Transfer the fish to a plate and set aside.
3. Return the skillet to the stove and add the butter.
4. Sauté the garlic until translucent, about 3 minutes.
5. Whisk in the flour to make a thick paste and cook, stirring constantly, until the mixture is golden brown, about 2 minutes.
6. Whisk in the chicken broth, lemon juice and zest.
7. Cook for about 4 minutes until the sauce is thickened.
8. Stir in the capers and serve the sauce over the fish.

Nutrition Info:
- Per Serving: Calories: 271;Fat: 13.0g;Protein: 30.0g;-Carbs: 7.0g.

Baked Haddock With Rosemary Gremolata

Servings:6
Cooking Time:35 Min + Marinating Time

Ingredients:
- 1 cup milk
- Salt and black pepper to taste
- 2 tbsp rosemary, chopped
- 1 garlic clove, minced
- 1 lemon, zested
- 1 ½ lb haddock fillets

Directions:
1. In a large bowl, coat the fish with milk, salt, pepper, and 1 tablespoon of rosemary. Refrigerate for 2 hours.
2. Preheat oven to 380 F. Carefully remove the haddock from the marinade, drain thoroughly, and place in a greased baking dish. Cover and bake 15–20 minutes until the fish is flaky. Remove fish from the oven and let it rest 5 minutes. To make the gremolata, mix the remaining rosemary, lemon zest, and garlic. Sprinkle the fish with gremolata and serve.

Nutrition Info:
- Per Serving: Calories: 112;Fat: 2g;Protein: 20g;Carbs: 3g.

Lemon-parsley Swordfish

Servings:4
Cooking Time: 17 To 20 Minutes

Ingredients:
- 1 cup fresh Italian parsley
- ¼ cup lemon juice
- ¼ cup extra-virgin olive oil
- ¼ cup fresh thyme
- 2 cloves garlic
- ½ teaspoon salt
- 4 swordfish steaks
- Olive oil spray

Directions:
1. Preheat the oven to 450ºF. Grease a large baking dish generously with olive oil spray.
2. Place the parsley, lemon juice, olive oil, thyme, garlic, and salt in a food processor and pulse until smoothly blended.
3. Arrange the swordfish steaks in the greased baking dish and spoon the parsley mixture over the top.
4. Bake in the preheated oven for 17 to 20 minutes until flaky.
5. Divide the fish among four plates and serve hot.

Nutrition Info:
- Per Serving: Calories: 396;Fat: 21.7g;Protein: 44.2g;Carbs: 2.9g.

Shrimp Quinoa Bowl With Black Olives

Servings:4
Cooking Time:20 Minutes

Ingredients:
- 10 black olives, pitted and halved
- ¼ cup olive oil
- 1 cup quinoa
- 1 lemon, cut in wedges
- 1 lb shrimp, peeled and cooked
- 2 tomatoes, sliced
- 2 bell peppers, thinly sliced
- 1 red onion, chopped
- 1 tsp dried dill
- 1 tbsp fresh parsley, chopped
- Salt and black pepper to taste

Directions:
1. Place the quinoa in a pot and cover with 2 cups of water over medium heat. Bring to a boil, reduce the heat, and simmer for 12-15 minutes or until tender. Remove from heat and fluff it with a fork. Mix in the quinoa with olive oil, dill, parsley, salt, and black pepper. Stir in tomatoes, bell peppers, olives, and onion. Serve decorated with shrimp and lemon wedges.

Nutrition Info:
- Per Serving: Calories: 662;Fat: 21g;Protein: 79g;Carbs: 38g.

Juicy Basil-tomato Scallops

Servings:4
Cooking Time:20 Minutes

Ingredients:
- 2 tbsp olive oil
- 1 tbsp basil, chopped
- 1 lb scallops, scrubbed
- 1 tbsp garlic, minced
- 1 onion, chopped
- 6 tomatoes, cubed
- 1 cup heavy cream
- 1 tbsp parsley, chopped

Directions:
1. Warm the olive oil in a skillet over medium heat and cook garlic and onion for 2 minutes. Stir in scallops, basil, tomatoes, heavy cream, and parsley and cook for an additional 7 minutes. Serve immediately.

Nutrition Info:
- Per Serving: Calories: 270;Fat: 12g;Protein: 11g;Carbs: 17g.

10-minute Cod With Parsley Pistou

Servings:4
Cooking Time: 10 Minutes

Ingredients:

- 1 cup packed roughly chopped fresh flat-leaf Italian parsley
- Zest and juice of 1 lemon
- 1 to 2 small garlic cloves, minced
- 1 teaspoon salt
- ½ teaspoon freshly ground black pepper
- 1 cup extra-virgin olive oil, divided
- 1 pound cod fillets, cut into 4 equal-sized pieces

Directions:

1. Make the pistou: Place the parsley, lemon zest and juice, garlic, salt, and pepper in a food processor until finely chopped.
2. With the food processor running, slowly drizzle in ¾ cup of olive oil until a thick sauce forms. Set aside.
3. Heat the remaining ¼ cup of olive oil in a large skillet over medium-high heat.
4. Add the cod fillets, cover, and cook each side for 4 to 5 minutes, until browned and cooked through.
5. Remove the cod fillets from the heat to a plate and top each with generous spoonfuls of the prepared pistou. Serve immediately.

Nutrition Info:

- Per Serving: Calories: 580;Fat: 54.6g;Protein: 21.1g;- Carbs: 2.8g.

Salmon & Celery Egg Bake

Servings:4
Cooking Time:40 Minutes

Ingredients:

- 2 tbsp olive oil
- 2 tbsp butter, melted
- 4 oz smoked salmon, flaked
- 1 cup cheddar cheese, grated
- 4 eggs, whisked
- ¼ cup plain yogurt
- 1 cup cream of celery soup
- 1 shallot, chopped
- 2 garlic cloves, minced
- ½ cup celery, chopped
- 8 slices fresh toast, cubed
- 1 tbsp mint leaves, chopped

Directions:

1. Preheat the oven to 360 F. In a bowl, mix eggs, yogurt, and celery soup. Warm olive oil in a skillet over medium heat and cook the shallot, garlic, and celery until tender. Place the toast cubes in a greased baking dish, top with cooked vegetables and salmon, and cover with egg mixture and butter. Bake for 22-25 minutes until it is cooked through. Scatter cheddar cheese on top and bake for another 5 minutes until the cheese melts. Serve garnished with mint leaves.

Nutrition Info:

- Per Serving: Calories: 392;Fat: 31g;Protein: 20g;Carbs: 9.6g.

Mackerel And Green Bean Salad

Servings:2
Cooking Time: 10 Minutes

Ingredients:

- 2 cups green beans
- 1 tablespoon avocado oil
- 2 mackerel fillets
- 4 cups mixed salad greens
- 2 hard-boiled eggs, sliced
- 1 avocado, sliced
- 2 tablespoons lemon juice
- 2 tablespoons olive oil
- 1 teaspoon Dijon mustard
- Salt and black pepper, to taste

Directions:

1. Cook the green beans in a medium saucepan of boiling water for about 3 minutes until crisp-tender. Drain and set aside.
2. Melt the avocado oil in a pan over medium heat. Add the mackerel fillets and cook each side for 4 minutes.
3. Divide the greens between two salad bowls. Top with the mackerel, sliced egg, and avocado slices.
4. In another bowl, whisk together the lemon juice, olive oil, mustard, salt, and pepper, and drizzle over the salad. Add the cooked green beans and toss to combine, then serve.

Nutrition Info:

- Per Serving: Calories: 737;Fat: 57.3g;Protein: 34.2g;- Carbs: 22.1g.

Baked Halibut With Eggplants

Servings:4
Cooking Time:35 Minutes

Ingredients:
- 2 tbsp olive oil
- ¼ cup tomato sauce
- 4 halibut fillets, boneless
- 2 eggplants, sliced
- Salt and black pepper to taste
- 2 tbsp balsamic vinegar
- 2 tbsp chives, chopped

Directions:
1. Preheat the oven to 380F. Warm the olive oil in a skillet over medium heat and fry the eggplant slices for 5-6 minutes, turning once; reserve. Add the tomato sauce, salt, pepper, and vinegar to the skillet and cook for 5 minutes. Return the eggplants to the skillet and cook for 2 minutes. Remove to a plate. Place the halibut fillets on a greased baking tray and bake for 12-15 minutes. Serve the halibut over the eggplants sprinkled with chives.

Nutrition Info:
- Per Serving: Calories: 300;Fat: 13g;Protein: 16g;Carbs: 19g.

Italian Canned Tuna & Bean Bowl

Servings:6
Cooking Time:30 Minutes

Ingredients:
- 3 tbsp olive oil
- 1 lb kale, chopped
- 1 onion, chopped
- 3 garlic cloves, minced
- 1 can sliced olives
- ¼ cup capers
- ¼ tsp red pepper flakes
- 2 cans tuna in olive oil
- 1 can cannellini beans
- ½ cup chicken broth
- Salt and black pepper to taste

Directions:
1. Steam the kale for approximately 4 minutes or until crisp-tender and set aside. Warm the olive oil in a saucepan over medium heat. Sauté the onion and garlic for 4 minutes, stirring often. Add the chicken broth, olives, capers, and crushed red pepper flakes and cook for 4-5 minutes, stirring often. Add the kale and stir. Remove to a bowl and mix in the tuna, beans, pepper, and salt. Serve and enjoy!

Nutrition Info:
- Per Serving: Calories: 636;Fat: 60g;Protein: 8g;Carbs: 22g.

Simple Salmon With Balsamic Haricots Vert

Servings:4
Cooking Time:25 Minutes

Ingredients:
- 2 tbsp olive oil
- 3 tbsp balsamic vinegar
- 1 garlic clove, minced
- ½ tsp red pepper flakes
- 1 ½ lb haricots vert, chopped
- Salt and black pepper to taste
- 1 red onion, sliced
- 4 salmon fillets, boneless

Directions:
1. Warm half of oil in a skillet over medium heat and sauté vinegar, onion, garlic, red pepper flakes, haricots vert, salt, and pepper for 6 minutes. Share into plates. Warm the remaining oil. Sprinkle salmon with salt and pepper and sear for 8 minutes on all sides. Serve with haricots vert.

Nutrition Info:
- Per Serving: Calories: 230;Fat: 16g;Protein: 17g;Carbs: 23g.

Shrimp & Squid Medley

Servings:4
Cooking Time:25 Minutes

Ingredients:
- 2 tbsp butter
- ½ lb squid rings
- 1 lb shrimp, peeled, deveined
- Salt and black pepper to taste
- 2 garlic cloves, minced
- 1 tsp rosemary, dried
- 1 red onion, chopped
- 1 cup vegetable stock
- 1 lemon, juiced
- 1 tbsp parsley, chopped

Directions:
1. Melt butter in a skillet over medium heat and cook onion and garlic for 4 minutes. Stir in shrimp, salt, pepper, squid rings, rosemary, vegetable stock, and lemon juice and bring to a boil. Simmer for 8 minutes. Put in parsley and serve.

Nutrition Info:
- Per Serving: Calories: 300;Fat: 14g;Protein: 7g;Carbs: 23g.

Seared Salmon With Lemon Cream Sauce

Servings:4
Cooking Time: 20 Minutes

Ingredients:
- 4 salmon fillets
- Sea salt and freshly ground black pepper, to taste
- 1 tablespoon extra-virgin olive oil
- ½ cup low-sodium vegetable broth
- Juice and zest of 1 lemon
- 1 teaspoon chopped fresh thyme
- ½ cup fat-free sour cream
- 1 teaspoon honey
- 1 tablespoon chopped fresh chives

Directions:
1. Preheat the oven to 400ºF.
2. Season the salmon lightly on both sides with salt and pepper.
3. Place a large ovenproof skillet over medium-high heat and add the olive oil.
4. Sear the salmon fillets on both sides until golden, about 3 minutes per side.
5. Transfer the salmon to a baking dish and bake in the preheated oven until just cooked through, about 10 minutes.
6. Meanwhile, whisk together the vegetable broth, lemon juice and zest, and thyme in a small saucepan over medium-high heat until the liquid reduces by about one-quarter, about 5 minutes.
7. Whisk in the sour cream and honey.
8. Stir in the chives and serve the sauce over the salmon.

Nutrition Info:
- Per Serving: Calories: 310;Fat: 18.0g;Protein: 29.0g;-Carbs: 6.0g.

Parchment Orange & Dill Salmon

Servings:4
Cooking Time:25 Minutes

Ingredients:
- 2 tbsp butter, melted
- 4 salmon fillets
- Salt and black pepper to taste
- 1 orange, juiced and zested
- 4 tbsp fresh dill, chopped

Directions:
1. Preheat oven to 375 F. Coat the salmon fillets on both sides with butter. Season with salt and pepper and divide them between 4 pieces of parchment paper. Drizzle the orange juice over each piece of fish and top with orange zest and dill. Wrap the paper around the fish to make packets. Place on a baking sheet and bake for 15-20 minutes until

the cod is cooked through. Serve and enjoy!

Nutrition Info:
- Per Serving: Calories: 481;Fat: 21g;Protein: 65g;Carbs: 4.2g.

Baked Salmon With Basil And Tomato

Servings:2
Cooking Time: 20 Minutes

Ingredients:
- 2 boneless salmon fillets
- 1 tablespoon dried basil
- 1 tomato, thinly sliced
- 1 tablespoon olive oil
- 2 tablespoons grated Parmesan cheese
- Nonstick cooking spray

Directions:
1. Preheat the oven to 375ºF. Line a baking sheet with a piece of aluminum foil and mist with nonstick cooking spray.
2. Arrange the salmon fillets onto the aluminum foil and scatter with basil. Place the tomato slices on top and drizzle with olive oil. Top with the grated Parmesan cheese.
3. Bake for about 20 minutes, or until the flesh is opaque and it flakes apart easily.
4. Remove from the oven and serve on a plate.

Nutrition Info:
- Per Serving: Calories: 403;Fat: 26.5g;Protein: 36.3g;-Carbs: 3.8g.

Parsley Tomato Tilapia

Servings:4
Cooking Time:20 Minutes

Ingredients:
- 2 tbsp olive oil
- 4 tilapia fillets, boneless
- ½ cup tomato sauce
- 2 tbsp parsley, chopped
- Salt and black pepper to taste

Directions:
1. Warm olive oil in a skillet over medium heat. Sprinkle tilapia with salt and pepper and cook until golden brown, flipping once, about 6 minutes. Pour in the tomato sauce and parsley and cook for an additional 4 minutes. Serve immediately.

Nutrition Info:
- Per Serving: Calories: 308;Fat: 17g;Protein: 16g;Carbs: 3g.

Trout Fillets With Horseradish Sauce

Servings:4
Cooking Time:35 Minutes

Ingredients:
- 3 tbsp olive oil
- 2 tbsp horseradish sauce
- 1 onion, sliced
- 2 tsp Italian seasoning
- 4 trout fillets, boneless
- ¼ cup panko breadcrumbs
- ½ cup green olives, pitted and chopped
- Salt and black pepper to taste
- 1 lemon, juiced

Directions:
1. Preheat the oven to 380F. Line a baking sheet with parchment paper. Sprinkle trout fillets with salt and pepper and dip in breadcrumbs. Arrange them along with the onion on the sheet. Sprinkle with olive oil, Italian seasoning, and lemon juice and bake for 15-18 minutes. Transfer to a serving plate and top with horseradish sauce and olives. Serve right away.

Nutrition Info:
- Per Serving: Calories: 310;Fat: 10g;Protein: 16g;Carbs: 25g.

Crispy Herb Crusted Halibut

Servings:4
Cooking Time: 20 Minutes

Ingredients:
- 4 halibut fillets, patted dry
- Extra-virgin olive oil, for brushing
- ½ cup coarsely ground unsalted pistachios
- 1 tablespoon chopped fresh parsley
- 1 teaspoon chopped fresh basil
- 1 teaspoon chopped fresh thyme
- Pinch sea salt
- Pinch freshly ground black pepper

Directions:
1. Preheat the oven to 350ºF. Line a baking sheet with parchment paper.
2. Place the fillets on the baking sheet and brush them generously with olive oil.
3. In a small bowl, stir together the pistachios, parsley, basil, thyme, salt, and pepper.
4. Spoon the nut mixture evenly on the fish, spreading it out so the tops of the fillets are covered.
5. Bake in the preheated oven until it flakes when pressed with a fork, about 20 minutes.
6. Serve immediately.

Nutrition Info:

- Per Serving: Calories: 262;Fat: 11.0g;Protein: 32.0g;-Carbs: 4.0g.

Avocado & Onion Tilapia

Servings:4
Cooking Time:10 Minutes

Ingredients:
- 1 tbsp olive oil
- 1 tbsp orange juice
- ¼ tsp kosher salt
- ½ tsp ground coriander seeds
- 4 tilapia fillets, skin-on
- ¼ cup chopped red onions
- 1 avocado, skinned and sliced

Directions:
1. In a bowl, mix together the olive oil, orange juice, ground coriander seeds, and salt. Add the fish and turn to coat on all sides. Arrange the fillets on a greased microwave-safe dish. Top with onion and cover the dish with plastic wrap, leaving a small part open at the edge to vent the steam. Microwave on high for about 3 minutes. The fish is done when it just begins to separate into chunks when pressed gently with a fork. Top the fillets with the avocado and serve.

Nutrition Info:
- Per Serving: Calories: 210;Fat: 11g;Protein: 25g;Carbs: 5g.

Thyme Hake With Potatoes

Servings:4
Cooking Time:40 Minutes

Ingredients:
- 1 ½ lb russet potatoes, unpeeled
- ¼ cup olive oil
- ½ tsp garlic powder
- ½ tsp paprika
- Salt and black pepper to taste
- 4 skinless hake fillets
- 4 fresh thyme sprigs
- 1 lemon, sliced

Directions:
1. Preheat oven to 425 F. Slice the potatoes and toss them with some olive oil, salt, pepper, paprika, and garlic powder in a bowl. Microwave for 12-14 minutes until potatoes are just tender, stirring halfway through microwaving.
2. Transfer the potatoes to a baking dish and press gently into an even layer. Season the hake with salt and pepper, and arrange it skinned side down over the potatoes. Drizzle with the remaining olive oil, then place thyme sprigs and lemon slices on top. Bake for 15-18 minutes until hake flakes apart when gently prodded with a paring knife. Serve

and enjoy!

Nutrition Info:
• Per Serving: Calories: 410;Fat: 16g;Protein: 34g;Carbs: 33g.

Lemon Trout With Roasted Beets

Servings:4
Cooking Time:45 Minutes

Ingredients:
• 1 lb medium beets, peeled and sliced
• 3 tbsp olive oil
• 4 trout fillets, boneless
• Salt and black pepper to taste
• 1 tbsp rosemary, chopped
• 2 spring onions, chopped
• 2 tbsp lemon juice
• ½ cup vegetable stock

Directions:
1. Preheat oven to 390F. Line a baking sheet with parchment paper. Arrange the beets on the sheet, season with salt and pepper, and drizzle with some olive oil. Roast for 20 minutes.
2. Warm the remaining oil in a skillet over medium heat. Cook trout fillets for 8 minutes on all sides; reserve. Add spring onions to the skillet and sauté for 2 minutes. Stir in lemon juice and stock and cook for 5-6 minutes until the sauce thickens. Remove the beets to a plate and top with trout fillets. Pour the sauce all over and sprinkle with rosemary.

Nutrition Info:
• Per Serving: Calories: 240;Fat: 6g;Protein: 18g;Carbs: 22g.

Parsley Salmon Bake

Servings:4
Cooking Time:20 Minutes

Ingredients:
• 2 tbsp olive oil
• 1 lb salmon fillets
• ¼ fresh parsley, chopped
• 1 garlic clove, minced
• ¼ tsp dried dill
• ¼ tsp chili powder
• ¼ tsp garlic powder
• 1 lemon, grated
• Salt and black pepper to taste

Directions:
1. Preheat oven to 350 F. Sprinkle the salmon with dill, chili powder, garlic powder, salt, and pepper.
2. Warm olive oil in a pan over medium heat and sear

salmon skin-side down for 5 minutes. Transfer to the oven and bake for another 4-5 minutes. Combine parsley, lemon zest, garlic, and salt in a bowl. Serve salmon topped with the mixture.

Nutrition Info:
• Per Serving: Calories: 212;Fat: 14g;Protein: 22g;Carbs: 0.5g.

Moules Mariniere (mussels In Wine Sauce)

Servings:4
Cooking Time:15 Minutes

Ingredients:
• 4 tbsp butter
• 4 lb cleaned mussels
• 2 cups dry white wine
• ½ tsp sea salt
• 6 garlic cloves, minced
• 1 shallot, diced
• ½ cup chopped parsley
• Juice of ½ lemon

Directions:
1. Pour the white wine, salt, garlic, shallots, and ¼ cup of the parsley into a large saucepan over medium heat. Cover and bring to boil. Add the mussels and simmer just until all of the mussels open, about 6 minutes. Do not overcook. With a slotted spoon, remove the mussels to a bowl. Add the butter and lemon juice to the saucepan, stir, and pour the broth over the mussels. Garnish with the remaining parsley and serve with a crusty, wholegrain baguette.

Nutrition Info:
• Per Serving: Calories: 528;Fat: 24g;Protein: 55g;Carbs: 20g.

Traditional Tuscan Scallops

Servings:4
Cooking Time:25 Minutes

Ingredients:
• 2 tbsp olive oil
• 1 lb sea scallops, rinsed
• 4 cups Tuscan kale
• 1 orange, juiced
• Salt and black pepper to taste
• ¼ tsp red pepper flakes

Directions:
1. Sprinkle scallops with salt and pepper.
2. Warm olive oil in a skillet over medium heat and brown scallops for 6-8 minutes on all sides. Remove to a plate and keep warm, covering with foil. In the same skillet, add the kale, red pepper flakes, orange juice, salt, and pepper and

cook until the kale wilts, about 4-5 minutes. Share the kale mixture into 4 plates and top with the scallops. Serve warm.

Nutrition Info:
• Per Serving: Calories: 214;Fat: 8g;Protein: 21g;Carbs: 15.2g.

Cheesy Smoked Salmon Crostini

Servings:4
Cooking Time:10 Min + Chilling Time

Ingredients:
• 4 oz smoked salmon, sliced
• 2 oz feta cheese, crumbled
• 4 oz cream cheese, softened
• 2 tbsp horseradish sauce
• 2 tsp orange zest
• 1 red onion, chopped
• 2 tbsp chives, chopped
• 1 baguette, sliced and toasted

Directions:
1. In a bowl, mix cream cheese, horseradish sauce, onion, feta cheese, and orange zest until smooth. Spread the mixture on the baguette slices. Top with salmon and chives to serve.

Nutrition Info:
• Per Serving: Calories: 290;Fat: 19g;Protein: 26g;Carbs: 5g.

White Wine Cod Fillets

Servings:4
Cooking Time:40 Minutes

Ingredients:
• 4 cod fillets
• Salt and black pepper to taste
• ½ fennel seeds, ground
• 1 tbsp olive oil
• ½ cup dry white wine
• ½ cup vegetable stock
• 2 garlic cloves, minced
• 1 tsp chopped fresh sage
• 4 rosemary sprigs

Directions:
1. Preheat oven to 375 F. Season the cod fillets with salt, pepper, and ground fennel seeds and place them in a greased baking dish. Add the wine, stock, garlic, and sage and drizzle with olive oil. Cover with foil and bake for 20 minutes until the fish flakes easily with a fork. Remove the fillets from the dish. Place the liquid in a saucepan over high heat and cook, stirring frequently, until reduced by half, about 10 minutes. Serve the fish topped with sauce and fresh rosemary sprigs.

Nutrition Info:
• Per Serving: Calories: 89;Fat: 0.6g;Protein: 18g;Carbs: 1.8g.

Cod Fettuccine

Servings:4
Cooking Time:30 Minutes

Ingredients:
• 1 lb cod fillets, cubed
• 16 oz fettuccine
• 3 tbsp olive oil
• 1 onion, finely chopped
• Salt and lemon pepper to taste
• 1 ½ cups heavy cream
• 1 cup Parmesan cheese, grated

Directions:
1. Boil salted water in a pot over medium heat and stir in fettuccine. Cook according to package directions and drain. Heat the olive oil in a large saucepan over medium heat and add the onion. Stir-fry for 3 minutes until tender. Sprinkle cod with salt and lemon pepper and add to saucepan; cook for 4–5 minutes until fish fillets and flakes easily with a fork. Stir in heavy cream for 2 minutes. Add in the pasta, tossing gently to combine. Cook for 3–4 minutes until sauce is slightly thickened. Sprinkle with Parmesan cheese.

Nutrition Info:
• Per Serving: Calories: 431;Fat: 36g;Protein: 42g;Carbs: 97g.

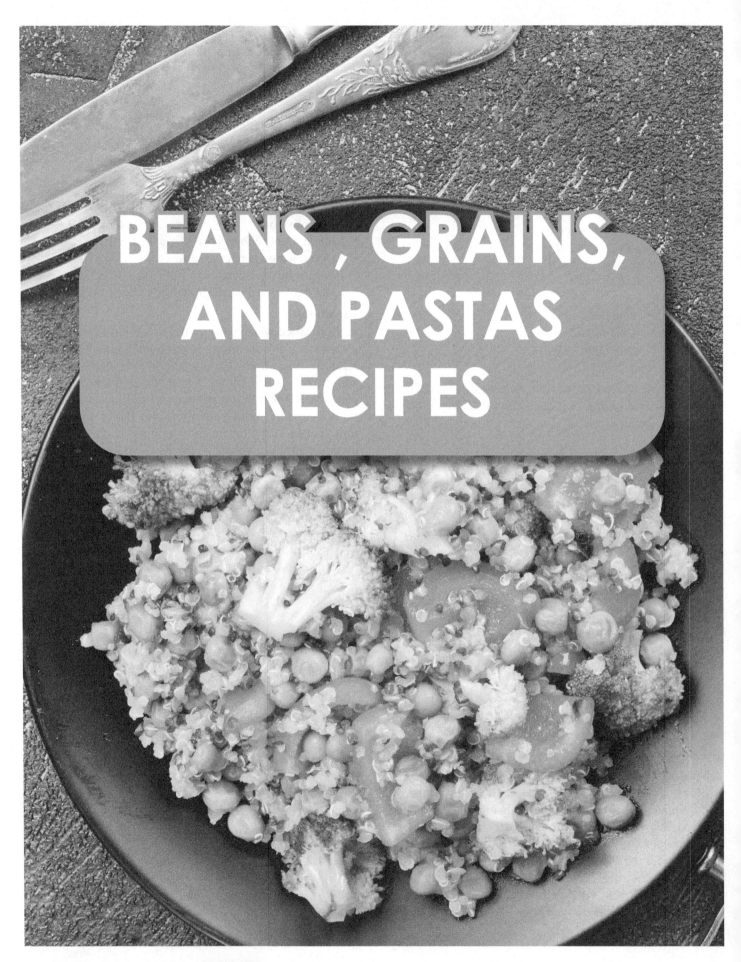

BEANS , GRAINS, AND PASTAS RECIPES

Beans , Grains, And Pastas Recipes

Ricotta & Olive Rigatoni

Servings:4
Cooking Time:25 Minutes

Ingredients:
- 2 tbsp extra-virgin olive oil
- 1 lb rigatoni
- ½ lb Ricotta cheese, crumbled
- ¾ cup black olives, chopped
- 10 sun-dried tomatoes, sliced
- 1 tbsp dried oregano
- Black pepper to taste

Directions:
1. Bring to a boil salted water in a pot over high heat. Add the rigatoni and cook according to package directions; drain. Heat the olive oil in a large saucepan over medium heat. Add the rigatoni, ricotta, olives, and sun-dried tomatoes. Toss mixture to combine and cook 2–3 minutes or until cheese just starts to melt. Season with oregano and pepper.

Nutrition Info:
- Per Serving: Calories: 383;Fat: 28g;Protein: 15g;Carbs: 21g.

Arrabbiata Penne Rigate

Servings:4
Cooking Time:30 Minutes

Ingredients:
- 2 tbsp olive oil
- 1 onion, chopped
- 6 cloves garlic, minced
- ½ red chili, chopped
- 2 cups canned tomatoes, diced
- ½ tsp sugar
- Salt and black pepper to taste
- 1 lb penne rigate
- 1 cup shredded mozzarella
- 1 cup fresh basil, chopped
- ½ cup grated Parmesan cheese

Directions:
1. Bring a large pot of salted water to a boil, add the penne, and cook for 7-9 minutes until al dente. Reserve ¼ cup pasta cooking water and drain pasta. Set aside.
2. Warm the oil in a saucepan over medium heat. Sauté the onion and garlic for 3-5 minutes or until softened. Add to-

matoes with their liquid, black pepper, sugar, and salt. Cook 20 minutes or until the sauce thickens. Add the pasta and reserved cooking water and stir for 2-3 minutes. Add mozzarella cheese and red chili and cook until the cheese melts, 3-4 minutes. Top with Parmesan and basil and serve.

Nutrition Info:
- Per Serving: Calories: 454;Fat: 12g;Protein: 18g;Carbs: 70g.

Bulgur Pilaf With Garbanzo

Servings:4
Cooking Time: 20 Minutes

Ingredients:
- 3 tablespoons extra-virgin olive oil
- 1 large onion, chopped
- 1 can garbanzo beans, rinsed and drained
- 2 cups bulgur wheat, rinsed and drained
- 1½ teaspoons salt
- ½ teaspoon cinnamon
- 4 cups water

Directions:
1. In a large pot over medium heat, heat the olive oil. Add the onion and cook for 5 minutes.
2. Add the garbanzo beans and cook for an additional 5 minutes.
3. Stir in the remaining ingredients.
4. Reduce the heat to low. Cover and cook for 10 minutes.
5. When done, fluff the pilaf with a fork. Cover and let sit for another 5 minutes before serving.

Nutrition Info:
- Per Serving: Calories: 462;Fat: 13.0g;Protein: 15.0g;-Carbs: 76.0g.

Rigatoni With Peppers & Mozzarella

Servings:4
Cooking Time:30 Min + Marinating Time

Ingredients:
- 1 lb fresh mozzarella cheese, cubed
- 3 tbsp olive oil
- ¼ cup chopped fresh chives
- ¼ cup basil, chopped
- ½ tsp red pepper flakes
- 1 tsp apple cider vinegar
- Salt and black pepper to taste

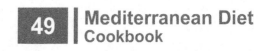

- 3 garlic cloves, minced
- 2 cups sliced onions
- 3 cups bell peppers, sliced
- 2 cups tomato sauce
- 8 oz rigatoni
- 1 tbsp butter
- ¼ cup grated Parmesan cheese

Directions:

1. Bring to a boil salted water in a pot over high heat. Add the rigatoni and cook according to package directions. Drain and set aside, reserving 1 cup of the cooking water. Combine the mozzarella, 1 tablespoon of olive oil, chives, basil, pepper flakes, apple cider vinegar, salt, and pepper. Let the cheese marinate for 30 minutes at room temperature.

2. Warm the remaining olive oil in a large skillet over medium heat. Stir-fry the garlic for 10 seconds and add the onions and peppers. Cook for 3-4 minutes, stirring occasionally until the onions are translucent. Pour in the tomato sauce, and reduce the heat to a simmer. Add the rigatoni and reserved cooking water and toss to coat. Heat off and adjust the seasoning with salt and pepper. Toss with marinated mozzarella cheese and butter. Sprinkle with Parmesan cheese and serve.

Nutrition Info:
- Per Serving: Calories: 434;Fat: 18g;Protein: 44g;Carbs: 27g.

Vegetable Lentils With Brown Rice

Servings:4
Cooking Time:40 Minutes

Ingredients:
- 1 ½ tbsp olive oil
- 2 ¼ cups vegetable broth
- ½ cup green lentils
- ½ cup brown rice
- ½ cup diced carrots
- ½ cup diced celery
- 1 can sliced olives
- ¼ cup diced red onion
- ¼ cup cilantro, chopped
- 1 tbsp lemon juice
- 1 garlic clove, minced
- Salt and black pepper to taste

Directions:

1. In a saucepan over high heat, bring the broth and lentils to a boil, cover, and lower the heat to medium-low. Cook for 8 minutes. Raise the heat to medium, and stir in the rice. Cover the pot and cook the mixture for 14 minutes or until the liquid is absorbed. Remove the pot from the heat and let sit covered for 2 minutes, then stir.

2. While the lentils and rice are cooking, combine carrots,

celery, olives, onion, and cilantro in a serving bowl. In a small bowl, whisk together the oil, lemon juice, garlic, salt, and black pepper. Set aside. Once the lentils and rice are done, add them to the serving bowl. Pour the dressing on top, and mix well. Serve warm.

Nutrition Info:
- Per Serving: Calories: 203;Fat: 7g;Protein: 10g;Carbs: 33g.

Tomato Sauce And Basil Pesto Fettuccine

Servings:4
Cooking Time: 15 Minutes

Ingredients:
- 4 Roma tomatoes, diced
- 2 teaspoons no-salt-added tomato paste
- 1 tablespoon chopped fresh oregano
- 2 garlic cloves, minced
- 1 cup low-sodium vegetable soup
- ½ teaspoon sea salt
- 1 packed cup fresh basil leaves
- ¼ cup pine nuts
- ¼ cup grated Parmesan cheese
- 2 tablespoons extra-virgin olive oil
- 1 pound cooked whole-grain fettuccine

Directions:

1. Put the tomatoes, tomato paste, oregano, garlic, vegetable soup, and salt in a skillet. Stir to mix well.

2. Cook over medium heat for 10 minutes or until lightly thickened.

3. Put the remaining ingredients, except for the fettuccine, in a food processor and pulse to combine until smooth.

4. Pour the puréed basil mixture into the tomato mixture, then add the fettuccine. Cook for a few minutes or until heated through and the fettuccine is well coated.

5. Serve immediately.

Nutrition Info:
- Per Serving: Calories: 389;Fat: 22.7g;Protein: 9.7g;Carbs: 40.2g.

Roasted Butternut Squash And Zucchini With Penne

Servings:6
Cooking Time: 30 Minutes

Ingredients:
- 1 large zucchini, diced
- 1 large butternut squash, peeled and diced
- 1 large yellow onion, chopped
- 2 tablespoons extra-virgin olive oil
- 1 teaspoon paprika

- ½ teaspoon garlic powder
- ½ teaspoon sea salt
- ½ teaspoon freshly ground black pepper
- 1 pound whole-grain penne
- ½ cup dry white wine
- 2 tablespoons grated Parmesan cheese

Directions:

1. Preheat the oven to 400ºF. Line a baking sheet with aluminum foil.
2. Combine the zucchini, butternut squash, and onion in a large bowl. Drizzle with olive oil and sprinkle with paprika, garlic powder, salt, and ground black pepper. Toss to coat well.
3. Spread the vegetables in the single layer on the baking sheet, then roast in the preheated oven for 25 minutes or until the vegetables are tender.
4. Meanwhile, bring a pot of water to a boil, then add the penne and cook for 14 minutes or until al dente. Drain the penne through a colander.
5. Transfer ½ cup of roasted vegetables in a food processor, then pour in the dry white wine. Pulse until smooth.
6. Pour the puréed vegetables in a nonstick skillet and cook with penne over medium-high heat for a few minutes to heat through.
7. Transfer the penne with the purée on a large serving plate, then spread the remaining roasted vegetables and Parmesan on top before serving.

Nutrition Info:
- Per Serving: Calories: 340;Fat: 6.2g;Protein: 8.0g;Carbs: 66.8g.

Classic Falafel

Servings:6
Cooking Time:20 Minutes

Ingredients:
- 2 cups olive oil
- Salt and black pepper to taste
- 1 cup chickpeas, soaked
- 5 scallions, chopped
- ¼ cup fresh parsley leaves
- ¼ cup fresh cilantro leaves
- ¼ cup fresh dill
- 6 garlic cloves, minced
- ½ tsp ground cumin
- ½ tsp ground coriander

Directions:

1. Pat dry chickpeas with paper towels and place them in your food processor. Add in scallions, parsley, cilantro, dill, garlic, salt, pepper, cumin, and ground coriander and pulse, scraping downsides of the bowl as needed. Shape the chickpea mixture into 2-tablespoon-size disks, about 1 ½ inches wide and 1 inch thick, and place on a parchment paper–lined baking sheet.
2. Warm the olive oil in a skillet over medium heat. Fry the falafel until deep golden brown, 2-3 minutes per side. With a slotted spoon, transfer falafel to a paper towel-lined plate to drain. Serve hot.

Nutrition Info:
- Per Serving: Calories: 349;Fat: 26.3g;Protein: 19g;Carbs: 9g.

Mediterranean Lentils

Servings:2
Cooking Time: 24 Minutes

Ingredients:
- 1 tablespoon olive oil
- 1 small sweet or yellow onion, diced
- 1 garlic clove, diced
- 1 teaspoon dried oregano
- ½ teaspoon ground cumin
- ½ teaspoon dried parsley
- ½ teaspoon salt, plus more as needed
- ¼ teaspoon freshly ground black pepper, plus more as needed
- 1 tomato, diced
- 1 cup brown or green lentils
- 2½ cups vegetable stock
- 1 bay leaf

Directions:

1. Set your Instant Pot to Sauté and heat the olive oil until it shimmers.
2. Add the onion and cook for 3 to 4 minutes until soft. Turn off the Instant Pot and add the garlic, oregano, cumin, parsley, salt, and pepper. Cook until fragrant, about 1 minute.
3. Stir in the tomato, lentils, stock, and bay leaf.
4. Lock the lid. Select the Manual mode and set the cooking time for 18 minutes at High Pressure.
5. When the timer beeps, perform a natural pressure release for 10 minutes, then release any remaining pressure. Carefully open the lid.
6. Remove and discard the bay leaf. Taste and season with more salt and pepper, as needed. If there's too much liquid remaining, select Sauté and cook until it evaporates.
7. Serve warm.

Nutrition Info:
- Per Serving: Calories: 426;Fat: 8.1g;Protein: 26.2g;Carbs: 63.8g.

Rice & Lentil Salad With Caramelized Onions

Servings:4
Cooking Time:1 Hour 15 Minutes

Ingredients:
- ¼ cup olive oil
- 2 cups lentils
- 1 cup brown rice
- 4 ½ cups water
- ½ tsp dried thyme
- ½ tsp dried tarragon
- 3 onions, peeled and sliced
- Salt and black pepper to taste

Directions:
1. Place the lentils and rice in a large saucepan with water. Bring to a boil, cover, and simmer for 23 minutes or until almost tender. Stir in the seasonings and cook for 25-30 minutes or until the rice is tender and the water is absorbed.
2. In a separate saucepan, warm the olive oil over medium heat. Add the onions and cook slowly, stirring frequently, until the onions brown and caramelize, for 17-20 minutes. Top with the caramelized onions. Serve and enjoy!

Nutrition Info:
- Per Serving: Calories: 498;Fat: 19g;Protein: 15g;Carbs: 63g.

Eggplant & Chickpea Casserole

Servings:6
Cooking Time:75 Minutes

Ingredients:
- ¼ cup olive oil
- 2 onions, chopped
- 1 green bell pepper, chopped
- Salt and black pepper to taste
- 3 garlic cloves, minced
- 1 tsp dried oregano
- ½ tsp ground cumin
- 1 lb eggplants, cubed
- 1 can tomatoes, diced
- 2 cans chickpeas

Directions:
1. Preheat oven to 400 F. Warm the olive oil in a skillet over medium heat. Add the onions, bell pepper, salt, and pepper.
2. Cook for about 5 minutes until softened. Stir in garlic, oregano, and cumin for about 30 seconds until fragrant. Transfer to a baking dish and add the eggplants, tomatoes, and chickpeas and stir. Place in the oven and bake for 45-60 minutes, shaking the dish twice during cooking. Serve.

Nutrition Info:

- Per Serving: Calories: 260;Fat: 12g;Protein: 8g;Carbs: 33.4g.

Ribollita (tuscan Bean Soup)

Servings:6
Cooking Time:1 Hour 45 Minutes

Ingredients:
- 3 tbsp olive oil
- Salt and black pepper to taste
- 2 cups canned cannellini beans
- 6 oz pancetta, chopped
- ¼ tsp red pepper flakes
- 1 onion, chopped
- 2 carrots, chopped
- 1 celery rib, chopped
- 3 garlic cloves, minced
- 4 cups chicken broth
- 1 lb lacinato kale, chopped
- 1 can diced tomatoes
- 1 rosemary sprig, chopped
- Crusty bread for serving

Directions:
1. Warm the olive oil in a skillet over medium heat and add the pancetta. Cook, stirring occasionally, until pancetta is lightly browned and fat has rendered, 5-6 minutes. Add onion, carrots, and celery and cook, stirring occasionally, until softened and lightly browned, 4-6 minutes. Stir in garlic and red pepper flakes and cook until fragrant, 1 minute.
2. Stir in broth, 2 cups of water, and beans and bring to a boil. Cover and simmer for 15 minutes. Stir in lacinato kale and tomatoes and cook for another 5 minutes. Sprinkle with rosemary and adjust the taste. Serve with crusty bread.

Nutrition Info:
- Per Serving: Calories: 385;Fat: 18g;Protein: 36g;Carbs: 25g.

Autumn Vegetable & Rigatoni Bake

Servings:6
Cooking Time:45 Minutes

Ingredients:
- 2 tbsp grated Pecorino-Romano cheese
- 2 tbsp olive oil
- 1 lb pumpkin, chopped
- 1 zucchini, chopped
- 1 onion, chopped
- 1 lb rigatoni
- Salt and black pepper to taste
- ½ tsp garlic powder
- ½ cup dry white wine

Directions:
1. Preheat oven to 420 F. Combine zucchini, pumpkin, on-

ion, and olive oil in a bowl. Arrange on a lined aluminum foil sheet and season with salt, pepper, and garlic powder. Bake for 30 minutes until tender. In a pot of boiling water, cook rigatoni for 8-10 minutes until al dente. Drain and set aside.

2. In a food processor, place ½ cup of the roasted veggies and wine and pulse until smooth. Transfer to a skillet over medium heat. Stir in rigatoni and cook until heated through. Top with the remaining vegetables and Pecorino cheese to serve.

Nutrition Info:
- Per Serving: Calories: 186;Fat: 11g;Protein: 10g;Carbs: 15g.

Authentic Fettuccine A La Puttanesca

Servings:4
Cooking Time:20 Minutes

Ingredients:
- 2 tbsp extra-virgin olive oil
- 20 Kalamata olives, chopped
- ¼ cup fresh basil, chopped
- 4 garlic cloves, minced
- 2 anchovy fillets, chopped
- ¼ tsp red pepper flakes
- 3 tbsp capers
- 3 cans diced tomatoes
- 8 oz fettuccine pasta
- 2 tbsp Parmesan cheese, grated
- Salt and black pepper to taste

Directions:
1. Cook the fettuccine pasta according to pack instructions, drain and let it to cool. Warm olive oil in a skillet over medium heat and cook garlic and red flakes for 2 minutes. Add in capers, anchovies, olives, salt, and pepper and cook for another 2-3 minutes until the anchovies melt into the oil. Blend tomatoes in a food processor. Pour into the skillet and stir-fry for 5 minutes. Mix in basil and pasta. Serve garnished with Parmesan cheese.

Nutrition Info:
- Per Serving: Calories: 443;Fat: 14g;Protein: 18g;Carbs: 65g.

Swoodles With Almond Butter Sauce

Servings:4
Cooking Time: 20 Minutes

Ingredients:
- Sauce:
- 1 garlic clove
- 1-inch piece fresh ginger, peeled and sliced
- ¼ cup chopped yellow onion
- ¾ cup almond butter

- 1 tablespoon tamari
- 1 tablespoon raw honey
- 1 teaspoon paprika
- 1 tablespoon fresh lemon juice
- ⅛ teaspoon ground red pepper
- Sea salt and ground black pepper, to taste
- ¼ cup water
- Swoodles:
- 2 large sweet potatoes, spiralized
- 2 tablespoons coconut oil, melted
- Sea salt and ground black pepper, to taste
- For Serving:
- ½ cup fresh parsley, chopped
- ½ cup thinly sliced scallions

Directions:
1. Make the Sauce
2. Put the garlic, ginger, and onion in a food processor, then pulse to combine well.
3. Add the almond butter, tamari, honey, paprika, lemon juice, ground red pepper, salt, and black pepper to the food processor. Pulse to combine well. Pour in the water during the pulsing until the mixture is thick and smooth.
4. Make the Swoodles:
5. Preheat the oven to 425ºF. Line a baking sheet with parchment paper.
6. Put the spiralized sweet potato in a bowl, then drizzle with olive oil. Toss to coat well. Transfer them on the baking sheet. Sprinkle with salt and pepper.
7. Bake in the preheated oven for 20 minutes or until lightly browned and al dente. Check the doneness during the baking and remove any well-cooked swoodles.
8. Transfer the swoodles on a large plate and spread with sauce, parsley, and scallions. Toss to serve.

Nutrition Info:
- Per Serving: Calories: 441;Fat: 33.6g;Protein: 12.0g;-Carbs: 29.6g.

Freekeh Pilaf With Dates And Pistachios

Servings:4
Cooking Time: 10 Minutes

Ingredients:
- 2 tablespoons extra-virgin olive oil, plus extra for drizzling
- 1 shallot, minced
- 1½ teaspoons grated fresh ginger
- ¼ teaspoon ground coriander
- ¼ teaspoon ground cumin
- Salt and pepper, to taste
- 1¾ cups water
- 1½ cups cracked freekeh, rinsed
- 3 ounces pitted dates, chopped

- ¼ cup shelled pistachios, toasted and coarsely chopped
- 1½ tablespoons lemon juice
- ¼ cup chopped fresh mint

Directions:

1. Set the Instant Pot to Sauté mode and heat the olive oil until shimmering.
2. Add the shallot, ginger, coriander, cumin, salt, and pepper to the pot and cook for about 2 minutes, or until the shallot is softened. Stir in the water and freekeh.
3. Secure the lid. Select the Manual mode and set the cooking time for 4 minutes at High Pressure. Once cooking is complete, do a quick pressure release. Carefully open the lid.
4. Add the dates, pistachios and lemon juice and gently fluff the freekeh with a fork to combine. Season to taste with salt and pepper.
5. Transfer to a serving dish and sprinkle with the mint. Serve drizzled with extra olive oil.

Nutrition Info:

- Per Serving: Calories: 280;Fat: 8.0g;Protein: 8.0g;Carbs: 46.0g.

Mozzarella & Asparagus Pasta

Servings:6
Cooking Time:40 Minutes

Ingredients:

- 1 ½ lb asparagus, trimmed, cut into 1-inch
- 2 tbsp olive oil
- 8 oz orecchiette
- 2 cups cherry tomatoes, halved
- Salt and black pepper to taste
- 2 cups fresh mozzarella, drained and chopped
- ⅓ cup torn basil leaves
- 2 tbsp balsamic vinegar

Directions:

1. Preheat oven to 390 F. In a large pot, cook the pasta according to the directions. Drain, reserving ¼ cup of cooking water.
2. In the meantime, in a large bowl, toss in asparagus, cherry tomatoes, oil, pepper, and salt. Spread the mixture onto a rimmed baking sheet and bake for 15 minutes, stirring twice throughout cooking. Remove the veggies from the oven, and add the cooked pasta to the baking sheet. Mix with a few tbsp of pasta water to smooth the sauce and veggies. Slowly mix in the mozzarella and basil. Drizzle with the balsamic vinegar and serve in bowls.

Nutrition Info:

- Per Serving: Calories: 188;Fat: 11g;Protein: 14g;Carbs: 23g.

Spaghetti With Pine Nuts And Cheese

Servings:4
Cooking Time: 11 Minutes

Ingredients:

- 8 ounces spaghetti
- 4 tablespoons almond butter
- 1 teaspoon freshly ground black pepper
- ½ cup pine nuts
- 1 cup fresh grated Parmesan cheese, divided

Directions:

1. Bring a large pot of salted water to a boil. Add the pasta and cook for 8 minutes.
2. In a large saucepan over medium heat, combine the butter, black pepper, and pine nuts. Cook for 2 to 3 minutes, or until the pine nuts are lightly toasted.
3. Reserve ½ cup of the pasta water. Drain the pasta and place it into the pan with the pine nuts.
4. Add ¾ cup of the Parmesan cheese and the reserved pasta water to the pasta and toss everything together to evenly coat the pasta.
5. Transfer the pasta to a serving dish and top with the remaining ¼ cup of the Parmesan cheese. Serve immediately.

Nutrition Info:

- Per Serving: Calories: 542;Fat: 32.0g;Protein: 20.0g;Carbs: 46.0g.

Genovese Mussel Linguine

Servings:4
Cooking Time:40 Minutes

Ingredients:

- 1 lb mussels, scrubbed and debearded
- 1 tbsp olive oil
- ½ cup Pinot Grigio wine
- 2 garlic cloves, minced
- ½ tsp red pepper flakes
- ½ lemon, zested and juiced
- 1 lb linguine
- Salt and black pepper to taste
- 2 tbsp parsley, finely chopped

Directions:

1. In a saucepan, bring mussels and wine to a boil, cover, and cook, shaking pan occasionally, until mussels open, 5-7 minutes. As they open, remove them with a slotted spoon into a bowl. Discard all closed mussels. Drain steaming liquid through fine-mesh strainer into a bowl, avoiding any gritty sediment that has settled on the bottom of the pan.
2. Wipe the pan clean. Warm the olive oil in the pan and stir-fry garlic and pepper flake until the garlic turn golden, 3 minutes. Stir in reserved mussel liquid and lemon zest and juice, bring to a simmer and cook for 3-4 minutes. Stir in

mussels and cook until heated through, 3 minutes.

3. Bring a large pot filled with salted water to a boil. Add pasta and cook until al dente. Reserve ½ cup of cooking liquid, drain pasta and return it to pot. Add the sauce and parsley and toss to combine and season to taste. Adjust consistency with the reserved cooking liquid as needed and serve.

Nutrition Info:
• Per Serving: Calories: 423;Fat: 9g;Protein: 16g;Carbs: 37g.

Cumin Quinoa Pilaf

Servings:2
Cooking Time: 5 Minutes

Ingredients:
• 2 tablespoons extra virgin olive oil
• 2 cloves garlic, minced
• 3 cups water
• 2 cups quinoa, rinsed
• 2 teaspoons ground cumin
• 2 teaspoons turmeric
• Salt, to taste
• 1 handful parsley, chopped

Directions:
1. Press the Sauté button to heat your Instant Pot.
2. Once hot, add the oil and garlic to the pot, stir and cook for 1 minute.
3. Add water, quinoa, cumin, turmeric, and salt, stirring well.
4. Lock the lid. Select the Manual mode and set the cooking time for 1 minute at High Pressure.
5. When the timer beeps, perform a natural pressure release for 10 minutes, then release any remaining pressure. Carefully remove the lid.
6. Fluff the quinoa with a fork. Season with more salt, if needed.
7. Sprinkle parsley on top and serve.

Nutrition Info:
• Per Serving: Calories: 384;Fat: 12.3g;Protein: 12.8g;-Carbs: 57.4g.

Valencian-style Mussel Rice

Servings:4
Cooking Time:40 Minutes

Ingredients:
• 1 lb mussels, cleaned and debearded
• 2 tbsp olive oil
• 2 garlic cloves, minced
• 1 yellow onion, chopped
• 2 tomatoes, chopped
• 2 cups fish stock
• 1 cup white rice
• 1 bunch parsley, chopped
• Salt and white pepper to taste

Directions:
1. Warm the olive oil in a pot over medium heat and cook onion and garlic for 5 minutes. Stir in rice for 1 minute. Pour in tomatoes and fish stock and bring to a boil. Add in the mussels and simmer for 20 minutes. Discard any unopened mussels. Adjust the taste with salt and white pepper. Serve topped with parsley.

Nutrition Info:
• Per Serving: Calories: 310;Fat: 15g;Protein: 12g;Carbs: 17g.

Slow Cooked Turkey And Brown Rice

Servings:6
Cooking Time: 3 Hours 10 Minutes

Ingredients:
• 1 tablespoon extra-virgin olive oil
• 1½ pounds ground turkey
• 2 tablespoons chopped fresh sage, divided
• 2 tablespoons chopped fresh thyme, divided
• 1 teaspoon sea salt
• ½ teaspoon ground black pepper
• 2 cups brown rice
• 1 can stewed tomatoes, with the juice
• ¼ cup pitted and sliced Kalamata olives
• 3 medium zucchini, sliced thinly
• ¼ cup chopped fresh flat-leaf parsley
• 1 medium yellow onion, chopped
• 1 tablespoon plus 1 teaspoon balsamic vinegar
• 2 cups low-sodium chicken stock
• 2 garlic cloves, minced
• ½ cup grated Parmesan cheese, for serving

Directions:
1. Heat the olive oil in a nonstick skillet over medium-high heat until shimmering.
2. Add the ground turkey and sprinkle with 1 tablespoon of sage, 1 tablespoon of thyme, salt and ground black pepper.
3. Sauté for 10 minutes or until the ground turkey is lightly browned.
4. Pour them in the slow cooker, then pour in the remaining ingredients, except for the Parmesan. Stir to mix well.
5. Put the lid on and cook on high for 3 hours or until the rice and vegetables are tender.
6. Pour them in a large serving bowl, then spread with Parmesan cheese before serving.

Nutrition Info:
• Per Serving: Calories: 499;Fat: 16.4g;Protein: 32.4g;-Carbs: 56.5g.

Marrakech-style Couscous

Servings:4
Cooking Time:25 Minutes

Ingredients:
- 2 tbsp olive oil
- 1 cup instant couscous
- 2 tbsp dried apricots, chopped
- 2 tbsp dried sultanas
- ½ onion, minced
- 1 orange, juiced and zested
- ¼ tsp paprika
- ¼ tsp turmeric
- ½ tsp garlic powder
- ½ tsp ground cumin
- ¼ tsp ground cinnamon
- Salt and black pepper to taste

Directions:
1. Warm olive oil in a pot over medium heat and sauté onion for 3 minutes. Add in orange juice, orange zest, garlic powder, cumin, salt, paprika, turmeric, cinnamon, black pepper, and 2 cups of water and bring to a boil. Stir in apricots, couscous, and sultanas. Remove from the heat and let sit covered for 5 minutes. Fluff the couscous using a fork. Serve.

Nutrition Info:
- Per Serving: Calories: 246;Fat: 7.4g;Protein: 5g;Carbs: 41.8g.

Bulgur Pilaf With Kale And Tomatoes

Servings:2
Cooking Time: 10 Minutes

Ingredients:
- 2 tablespoons olive oil
- 2 cloves garlic, minced
- 1 bunch kale, trimmed and cut into bite-sized pieces
- Juice of 1 lemon
- 2 cups cooked bulgur wheat
- 1 pint cherry tomatoes, halved
- Sea salt and freshly ground pepper, to taste

Directions:
1. Heat the olive oil in a large skillet over medium heat. Add the garlic and sauté for 1 minute.
2. Add the kale leaves and stir to coat. Cook for 5 minutes until leaves are cooked through and thoroughly wilted.
3. Add the lemon juice, bulgur and tomatoes. Season with sea salt and freshly ground pepper to taste, then serve.

Nutrition Info:
- Per Serving: Calories: 300;Fat: 14.0g;Protein: 6.2g;Carbs: 37.8g.

Brown Rice Pilaf With Pistachios And Raisins

Servings:6
Cooking Time: 15 Minutes

Ingredients:
- 1 tablespoon extra-virgin olive oil
- 1 cup chopped onion
- ½ cup shredded carrot
- ½ teaspoon ground cinnamon
- 1 teaspoon ground cumin
- 2 cups brown rice
- 1¾ cups pure orange juice
- ¼ cup water
- ½ cup shelled pistachios
- 1 cup golden raisins
- ½ cup chopped fresh chives

Directions:
1. Heat the olive oil in a saucepan over medium-high heat until shimmering.
2. Add the onion and sauté for 5 minutes or until translucent.
3. Add the carrots, cinnamon, and cumin, then sauté for 1 minutes or until aromatic.
4. Pour int the brown rice, orange juice, and water. Bring to a boil. Reduce the heat to medium-low and simmer for 7 minutes or until the liquid is almost absorbed.
5. Transfer the rice mixture in a large serving bowl, then spread with pistachios, raisins, and chives. Serve immediately.

Nutrition Info:
- Per Serving: Calories: 264;Fat: 7.1g;Protein: 5.2g;Carbs: 48.9g.

Spinach & Salmon Fettuccine In White Sauce

Servings:4
Cooking Time:35 Minutes

Ingredients:
- 5 tbsp butter
- 16 oz fettuccine
- 4 salmon fillets, cubed
- Salt and black pepper to taste
- 3 garlic cloves, minced
- 1 ¼ cups heavy cream
- ½ cup dry white wine
- 1 tsp grated lemon zest
- 1 cup baby spinach
- Lemon wedges for garnishing

Directions:
1. In a pot of boiling water, cook the fettuccine pasta for

8-10 minutes until al dente. Drain and set aside.
2. Melt half of the butter in a large skillet; season the salmon with salt, black pepper, and cook in the butter until golden brown on all sides and flaky within, 8 minutes. Transfer to a plate and set aside.
3. Add the remaining butter to the skillet to melt and stir in the garlic. Cook until fragrant, 1 minute. Mix in heavy cream, white wine, lemon zest, salt, and pepper. Allow boiling over low heat for 5 minutes. Stir in spinach, allow wilting for 2 minutes and stir in fettuccine and salmon until well-coated in the sauce. Garnish with lemon wedges.

Nutrition Info:
• Per Serving: Calories: 795;Fat: 46g;Protein: 72g;Carbs: 20g.

Mustard Vegetable Millet

Servings:6
Cooking Time:35 Minutes

Ingredients:
• 6 oz okra, cut into 1-inch lengths
• 3 tbsp olive oil
• 6 oz asparagus, chopped
• Salt and black pepper to taste
• 1 ½ cups whole millet
• 2 tbsp lemon juice
• 2 tbsp minced shallot
• 1 tsp Dijon mustard
• 6 oz cherry tomatoes, halved
• 3 tbsp chopped fresh dill
• 2 oz goat cheese, crumbled

Directions:
1. In a large pot, bring 4 quarts of water to a boil. Add asparagus, snap peas, and salt and cook until crisp-tender, about 3 minutes. Using a slotted spoon, transfer vegetables to a large plate and let cool completely, about 15 minutes. Add millet to water, return to a boil, and cook until grains are tender, 15-20 minutes.
2. Drain millet, spread in rimmed baking sheet, and let cool completely, 15 minutes. Whisk oil, lemon juice, shallot, mustard, salt, and pepper in a large bowl. Add vegetables, millet, tomatoes, dill, and half of the goat cheese and toss gently to combine. Season with salt and pepper. Sprinkle with remaining goat cheese to serve.

Nutrition Info:
• Per Serving: Calories: 315;Fat: 19g;Protein: 13g;Carbs: 35g.

Cheesy Sage Farro

Servings:4
Cooking Time:50 Minutes

Ingredients:
• 2 tbsp olive oil
• 1 cup farro
• 1 red onion, chopped
• 5 sage leaves
• 1 garlic clove, minced
• 1 tbsp Parmesan cheese, grated
• 6 cups veggie stock
• Salt and black pepper to taste

Directions:
1. Warm the olive oil in a skillet over medium heat and cook onion and garlic for 5 minutes. Stir in sage leaves, faro, veggie stock, salt, and pepper and bring to a simmer. Cook for 40 minutes. Mix in Parmesan cheese and serve.

Nutrition Info:
• Per Serving: Calories: 220;Fat: 7.1g;Protein: 4g;Carbs: 8.9g.

Arugula & Cheese Pasta With Red Sauce

Servings:6
Cooking Time:60 Minutes

Ingredients:
• ¼ cup olive oil
• 1 shallot, sliced thin
• 2 lb cherry tomatoes, halved
• 3 large garlic cloves, sliced
• 1 tbsp red wine vinegar
• 3 oz ricotta cheese, crumbled
• 1 tsp sugar
• Salt and black pepper to taste
• ¼ tsp red pepper flakes
• 1 lb penne
• 4 oz baby arugula

Directions:
1. Preheat oven to 350 F. Toss shallot with 1 tsp of oil in a bowl. In a separate bowl, toss tomatoes with remaining oil, garlic, vinegar, sugar, salt, pepper, and flakes. Spread tomato mixture in even layer in rimmed baking sheet, scatter shallot over tomatoes, and roast until edges of shallot begin to brown and tomato skins are slightly charred, 35-40 minutes; do not stir. Let cool for 5 to 10 minutes.
2. Meanwhile, bring a pot filled with salted water to a boil and add pasta. Cook, stirring often until al dente. Reserve ½ cup cooking water, then drain pasta and return it to pot. Add arugula to pasta and toss until wilted. Using a spatula, scrape tomato mixture onto pasta and toss to combine. Sea-

son to taste and adjust consistency with reserved cooking water as needed. Serve, passing ricotta cheese separately.

Nutrition Info:
- Per Serving: Calories: 444;Fat: 19g;Protein: 18g;Carbs: 44g.

Cherry Tomato Cannellini Beans

Servings:4
Cooking Time:10 Minutes

Ingredients:
- 2 tbsp olive oil
- 15 oz canned cannellini beans
- 10 cherry tomatoes, halved
- 2 spring onions, chopped
- 1 tsp paprika
- Salt and black pepper to taste
- ½ tsp ground cumin
- 1 tbsp lime juice

Directions:
1. Place beans, cherry tomatoes, spring onions, olive oil, paprika, salt, pepper, cumin, and lime juice in a bowl and toss to combine. Transfer to the fridge for 10 minutes. Serve.

Nutrition Info:
- Per Serving: Calories: 300;Fat: 8g;Protein: 13g;Carbs: 26g.

Mint Brown Rice

Servings:2
Cooking Time: 22 Minutes

Ingredients:
- 2 cloves garlic, minced
- ¼ cup chopped fresh mint, plus more for garnish
- 1 tablespoon chopped dried chives
- 1 cup short- or long-grain brown rice
- 1½ cups water or low-sodium vegetable broth
- ½ to 1 teaspoon sea salt

Directions:
1. Place the garlic, mint, chives, rice, and water in the Instant Pot. Stir to combine.
2. Secure the lid. Select the Manual mode and set the cooking time for 22 minutes at High Pressure.
3. Once cooking is complete, do a natural pressure release for 10 minutes, then release any remaining pressure. Carefully open the lid.
4. Add salt to taste. Serve garnished with more mint.

Nutrition Info:
- Per Serving: Calories: 514;Fat: 6.6g;Protein: 20.7g;-Carbs: 80.4g.

Old-fashioned Pasta Primavera

Servings:4
Cooking Time:25 Minutes

Ingredients:
- ½ cup grated Pecorino Romano cheese
- 2 cups cauliflower florets, cut into matchsticks
- ¼ cup olive oil
- 16 oz tortiglioni
- ½ cup chopped green onions
- 1 red bell pepper, sliced
- 4 garlic cloves, minced
- 1 cup grape tomatoes, halved
- 2 tsp dried Italian seasoning
- ½ lemon, juiced

Directions:
1. In a pot of boiling water, cook the tortiglioni pasta for 8-10 minutes until al dente. Drain and set aside.
2. Heat olive oil in a skillet and sauté onion, cauliflower, and bell pepper for 7 minutes. Mix in garlic and cook until fragrant, 30 seconds. Stir in the tomatoes and Italian seasoning; cook until the tomatoes soften, 5 minutes. Mix in the lemon juice and tortiglioni. Garnish with cheese.

Nutrition Info:
- Per Serving: Calories: 283;Fat: 18g;Protein: 15g;Carbs: 5g.

Leftover Pasta & Mushroom Frittata

Servings:4
Cooking Time:25 Minutes

Ingredients:
- 2 tbsp olive oil
- 4 oz leftover spaghetti, cooked
- 8 large eggs, beaten
- ¼ cup heavy cream
- ½ tsp Italian seasoning
- ½ tsp garlic salt
- 1/8 tsp garlic pepper
- 1 cup chopped mushrooms
- 1 cup Pecorino cheese, grated

Directions:
1. Preheat your broiler. Warm the olive oil in a large skillet over medium heat. Add mushrooms and cook for 3–4 minutes, until almost tender. In a large bowl, beat the eggs with cream, Italian seasoning, garlic salt, and garlic pepper. Stir in the leftover spaghetti. Pour the egg mixture over the mushrooms and level with a spatula. Cook for 5–7 minutes until the eggs are almost set. Sprinkle with cheese and place under broiler for 3–5 minutes, until the cheese melts. Serve.

Nutrition Info:
- Per Serving: Calories: 400;Fat: 30g;Protein: 23g;Carbs: 11g.

Pork & Garbanzo Cassoulet

Servings:4
Cooking Time:50 Minutes

Ingredients:
- 2 tbsp olive oil
- 2 lb pork stew meat, cubed
- 1 leek, chopped
- 1 red bell pepper, chopped
- 3 garlic cloves, minced
- 2 tsp sage
- 4 oz canned garbanzo beans
- 1 cup chicken stock
- 2 zucchinis, chopped
- 2 tbsp tomato paste
- 2 tbsp parsley, chopped

Directions:
1. Warm the olive oil in a pot over medium heat and sear pork meat for 10 minutes, stirring occasionally. Add in leek, bell pepper, garlic, and zucchini and sauté for 5 minutes. Stir in tomato paste and sage for 1 minute and pour in garbanzo beans and chicken stock. Cover and bring to a boil, then reduce the heat and simmer for 30 minutes. Adjust the seasoning and serve garnished with parsley.

Nutrition Info:
- Per Serving: Calories: 430;Fat: 16g;Protein: 44g;Carbs: 28g.

Rich Cauliflower Alfredo

Servings:4
Cooking Time: 30 Minutes

Ingredients:
- Cauliflower Alfredo Sauce:
- 1 tablespoon avocado oil
- ½ yellow onion, diced
- 2 cups cauliflower florets
- 2 garlic cloves, minced
- 1½ teaspoons miso
- 1 teaspoon Dijon mustard
- Pinch of ground nutmeg
- ½ cup unsweetened almond milk
- 1½ tablespoons fresh lemon juice
- 2 tablespoons nutritional yeast
- Sea salt and ground black pepper, to taste
- Fettuccine:
- 1 tablespoon avocado oil
- ½ yellow onion, diced
- 1 cup broccoli florets
- 1 zucchini, halved lengthwise and cut into ¼-inch-thick half-moons
- Sea salt and ground black pepper, to taste
- ½ cup sun-dried tomatoes, drained if packed in oil
- 8 ounces cooked whole-wheat fettuccine

- ½ cup fresh basil, cut into ribbons

Directions:
1. Make the Sauce:
2. Heat the avocado oil in a nonstick skillet over medium-high heat until shimmering.
3. Add half of the onion to the skillet and sauté for 5 minutes or until translucent.
4. Add the cauliflower and garlic to the skillet. Reduce the heat to low and cook for 8 minutes or until the cauliflower is tender.
5. Pour them in a food processor, add the remaining ingredients for the sauce and pulse to combine well. Set aside.
6. Make the Fettuccine:
7. Heat the avocado oil in a nonstick skillet over medium-high heat.
8. Add the remaining half of onion and sauté for 5 minutes or until translucent.
9. Add the broccoli and zucchini. Sprinkle with salt and ground black pepper, then sauté for 5 minutes or until tender.
10. Add the sun-dried tomatoes, reserved sauce, and fettuccine. Sauté for 3 minutes or until well-coated and heated through.
11. Serve the fettuccine on a large plate and spread with basil before serving.

Nutrition Info:
- Per Serving: Calories: 288;Fat: 15.9g;Protein: 10.1g;-Carbs: 32.5g.

Apricot & Almond Couscous

Servings:4
Cooking Time:25 Minutes

Ingredients:
- 2 tbsp olive oil
- 1 small onion, diced
- 1 cup couscous
- 2 cups water
- ½ cup dried apricots, soaked
- ½ cup slivered hazelnuts
- ½ tsp dried mint
- ½ tsp dried thyme

Directions:
1. In a skillet, heat the olive and stir-fry the onion until translucent and soft. Stir in the couscous and cook for 2-3 minutes. Add the water, cover, and cook for 8-10 minutes until the water is mostly absorbed. Remove from the heat and let sit for a few minutes. Fluff with a fork and fold in the apricots, nuts, mint, and thyme.

Nutrition Info:
- Per Serving: Calories: 388;Fat: 8g;Protein: 14g;Carbs: 36g.

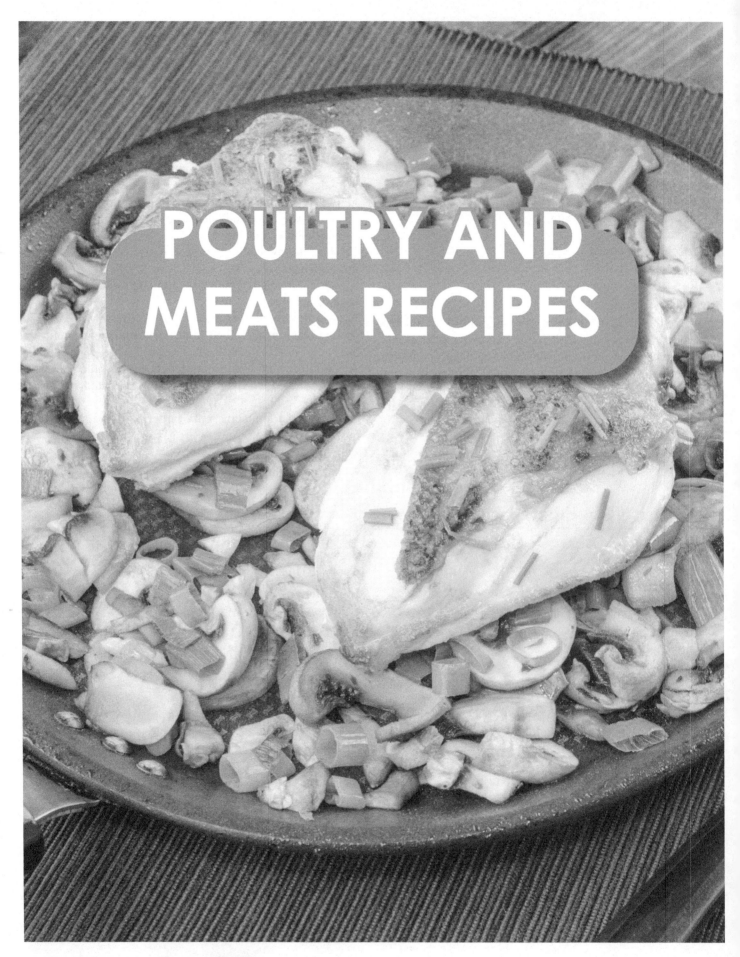

POULTRY AND MEATS RECIPES

Poultry And Meats Recipes

Italian Potato & Chicken

Servings:4
Cooking Time:50 Minutes

Ingredients:
- 3 tbsp canola oil
- 1 lb chicken breasts, halved
- Salt and black pepper to taste
- 2 garlic cloves, minced
- 2 shallots, chopped
- 1 lb red potatoes, sliced
- 3 tomatoes, chopped
- ¼ cup chicken stock
- 1 tbsp Italian seasoning

Directions:
1. Warm the canola oil in a skillet over medium heat and cook chicken, garlic, salt, and pepper for 6 minutes on both sides. Stir in shallots, potatoes, tomatoes, stock, and Italian seasoning and bring to a boil. Cook for 30 minutes. Serve.

Nutrition Info:
- Per Serving: Calories: 320;Fat: 13g;Protein: 16g;Carbs: 25g.

Balsamic Chicken Breasts With Feta

Servings:4
Cooking Time:35 Minutes

Ingredients:
- 1 lb chicken breasts, cut into strips
- 2 tbsp olive oil
- 1 fennel bulb, chopped
- Salt and black pepper to taste
- 2 tbsp balsamic vinegar
- 2 cups tomatoes, cubed
- 1 tbsp chives, chopped
- ¼ cup feta cheese, crumbled

Directions:
1. Warm the olive oil in a skillet over medium heat and sear chicken for 5 minutes, stirring often. Mix in fennel, salt, pepper, vinegar, and tomatoes and cook for 20 minutes. Top with feta cheese and chives and serve.

Nutrition Info:
- Per Serving: Calories: 290;Fat: 16g;Protein: 15g;Carbs: 16g.

Rich Pork In Cilantro Sauce

Servings:4
Cooking Time:30 Minutes

Ingredients:
- ½ cup olive oil
- 1 lb pork stew meat, cubed
- 1 tbsp walnuts, chopped
- 2 tbsp cilantro, chopped
- 2 tbsp basil, chopped
- 2 garlic cloves, minced
- Salt and black pepper to taste
- 2 cups Greek yogurt

Directions:
1. In a food processor, blend cilantro, basil, garlic, walnuts, yogurt, salt, pepper, and half of the oil until smooth.
2. Warm the remaining oil in a skillet over medium heat. Brown pork meat for 5 minutes. Pour sauce over meat and bring to a boil. Cook for another 15 minutes. Serve.

Nutrition Info:
- Per Serving: Calories: 280;Fat: 12g;Protein: 19g;Carbs: 21g.

Rosemary Tomato Chicken

Servings:4
Cooking Time:50 Minutes

Ingredients:
- 2 tbsp olive oil
- 1 lb chicken breasts, sliced
- 1 onion, chopped
- 1 carrot, chopped
- 2 garlic cloves, minced
- ½ cup chicken stock
- 1 tsp oregano, dried
- 1 tsp tarragon, dried
- 1 tsp rosemary, dried
- 1 cup canned tomatoes, diced
- Salt and black pepper to taste

Directions:
1. Warm the olive oil in a pot over medium heat and cook the chicken for 8 minutes on both sides. Put in carrot, garlic, and onion and cook for an additional 3 minutes. Season with salt and pepper. Pour in stock, oregano, tarragon, rosemary, and tomatoes and bring to a boil; simmer for 25 minutes. Serve.

Nutrition Info:
- Per Serving: Calories: 260;Fat: 12g;Protein: 10g;Carbs: 16g.

Baked Chicken & Veggie

Servings:4
Cooking Time:50 Minutes

Ingredients:
- 4 fresh prunes, cored and quartered
- 2 tbsp olive oil
- 4 chicken legs
- 1 lb baby potatoes, halved
- 1 carrot, julienned
- 2 tbsp chopped fresh parsley
- Salt and black pepper to taste

Directions:
1. Preheat oven to 420 F. Combine potatoes, carrot, prunes, olive oil, salt, and pepper in a bowl. Transfer to a baking dish. Top with chicken. Season with salt and pepper. Roast for about 40-45 minutes. Serve topped with parsley.

Nutrition Info:
- Per Serving: Calories: 473;Fat: 23g;Protein: 21g;Carbs: 49g.

Cilantro Turkey Penne With Asparagus

Servings:4
Cooking Time:40 Minutes

Ingredients:
- 3 tbsp olive oil
- 16 oz penne pasta
- 1 lb turkey breast strips
- 1 lb asparagus, chopped
- 1 tsp basil, chopped
- Salt and black pepper to taste
- ½ cup tomato sauce
- 2 tbsp cilantro, chopped

Directions:
1. Bring to a boil salted water in a pot over medium heat and cook penne until "al dente", 8-10 minutes. Drain and set aside; reserve 1 cup of the cooking water.
2. Warm the olive oil in a skillet over medium heat and sear turkey for 4 minutes, stirring periodically. Add in asparagus and sauté for 3-4 more minutes. Pour in the tomato sauce and reserved pasta liquid and bring to a boil; simmer for 20 minutes. Stir in cooked penne, season with salt and pepper, and top with the basil and cilantro to serve.

Nutrition Info:
- Per Serving: Calories: 350;Fat: 22g;Protein: 19g;Carbs: 23g.

Provençal Flank Steak Au Pistou

Servings:4
Cooking Time:25 Minutes

Ingredients:
- 8 tbsp olive oil
- 1 lb flank steak
- Salt and black pepper to taste
- ½ cup parsley, chopped
- ¼ cup fresh basil, chopped
- 2 garlic cloves, minced
- ½ tsp celery seeds
- 1 orange, zested and juiced
- 1 tsp red pepper flakes
- 1 tbsp red wine vinegar

Directions:
1. Place the parsley, basil, garlic, orange zest and juice, celery seeds, salt, pepper, and red pepper flakes, and pulse until finely chopped in your food processor. With the processor running, stream in the red wine vinegar and 6 tbsp of olive oil until well combined. Set aside until ready to serve.
2. Preheat your grill. Rub the steak with the remaining olive oil, salt, and pepper. Place the steak on the grill and cook for 6-8 minutes on each side. Remove and leave to sit for 10 minutes. Slice the steak and drizzle with pistou. Serve.

Nutrition Info:
- Per Serving: Calories: 441;Fat: 36g;Protein: 25g;Carbs: 3g.

Paprika Chicken With Caper Dressing

Servings:4
Cooking Time:35 Minutes

Ingredients:
- 2 tbsp canola oil
- 4 chicken breast halves
- Salt and black pepper to taste
- 1 tbsp sweet paprika
- 1 onion, chopped
- 1 tbsp balsamic vinegar
- 2 tbsp parsley, chopped
- 1 avocado, peeled and cubed
- 2 tbsp capers

Directions:
1. Preheat the grill over medium heat. Rub chicken halves with half of the canola oil, paprika, salt, and pepper and grill them for 14 minutes on both sides. Share into plates. Combine onion, remaining oil, vinegar, parsley, avocado, and capers in a bowl. Pour the sauce over the chicken and serve.

Nutrition Info:

- Per Serving: Calories: 300;Fat: 13g;Protein: 15g;Carbs: 25g.

Sweet Chicken Stew

Servings:4
Cooking Time:50 Minutes

Ingredients:
- 2 tbsp olive oil
- 3 garlic cloves, minced
- 3 tbsp cilantro, chopped
- Salt and black pepper to taste
- 2 cups chicken stock
- 2 shallots, thinly sliced
- 1 lb chicken breasts, cubed
- 5 oz dried pitted prunes, halved

Directions:
1. Warm the olive oil in a pot over medium heat and cook shallots and garlic for 3 minutes. Add in chicken breasts and cook for another 5 minutes, stirring occasionally. Pour in chicken stock and prunes and season with salt and pepper. Cook for 30 minutes. Garnish with cilantro and serve.

Nutrition Info:
- Per Serving: Calories: 310;Fat: 26g;Protein: 7g;Carbs: 16g.

Slow Cooker Beef With Tomatoes

Servings:4
Cooking Time:8 Hours 10 Minutes

Ingredients:
- 1 ½ lb beef shoulder, cubed
- ½ cup chicken stock
- 2 tomatoes, chopped
- 2 garlic cloves, minced
- 1 tbsp cinnamon powder
- Salt and black pepper to taste
- 2 tbsp cilantro, chopped

Directions:
1. Place the beef, tomatoes, garlic, cinnamon, salt, pepper, chicken stock, and cilantro in your slow cooker. Cover with the lid and cook for 8 hours on Low. Serve immediately.

Nutrition Info:
- Per Serving: Calories: 360;Fat: 16g;Protein: 16g;Carbs: 19g.

Chermoula Roasted Pork Tenderloin

Servings:2
Cooking Time: 20 Minutes

Ingredients:
- ½ cup fresh cilantro

- ½ cup fresh parsley
- 6 small garlic cloves
- 3 tablespoons olive oil, divided
- 3 tablespoons freshly squeezed lemon juice
- 2 teaspoons cumin
- 1 teaspoon smoked paprika
- ½ teaspoon salt, divided
- Pinch freshly ground black pepper
- 1 pork tenderloin

Directions:
1. Preheat the oven to 425ºF.
2. In a food processor, combine the cilantro, parsley, garlic, 2 tablespoons of olive oil, lemon juice, cumin, paprika, and ¼ teaspoon of salt. Pulse 15 to 20 times, or until the mixture is fairly smooth. Scrape the sides down as needed to incorporate all the ingredients. Transfer the sauce to a small bowl and set aside.
3. Season the pork tenderloin on all sides with the remaining ¼ teaspoon of salt and a generous pinch of black pepper.
4. Heat the remaining 1 tablespoon of olive oil in a sauté pan.
5. Sear the pork for 3 minutes, turning often, until golden brown on all sides.
6. Transfer the pork to a baking dish and roast in the preheated oven for 15 minutes, or until the internal temperature registers 145ºF.
7. Cool for 5 minutes before serving.

Nutrition Info:
- Per Serving: Calories: 169;Fat: 13.1g;Protein: 11.0g;-Carbs: 2.9g.

Spinach-ricotta Chicken Rolls

Servings:4
Cooking Time:55 Minutes

Ingredients:
- 2 tbsp olive oil
- 4 chicken breast halves
- 1 lb baby spinach
- 2 garlic cloves, minced
- 1 lemon, zested
- ½ cup crumbled ricotta cheese
- 1 tbsp pine nuts, toasted
- Salt and black pepper to taste

Directions:
1. Preheat oven to 350 F. Pound the chicken breasts to ½-inch thickness with a meat mallet and season with salt and pepper.
2. Warm olive oil in a pan over medium heat and sauté spinach for 4-5 minutes until it wilts. Stir in garlic, salt, lemon zest, and pepper for 20-30 seconds. Let cool slightly and add in ricotta cheese and pine nuts; mix well. Spoon the

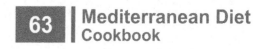

mixture over the chicken breasts, wrap around the filling, and secure the ends with toothpicks. Arrange the breasts on a greased baking dish and bake for 35-40 minutes. Let sit for a few minutes and slice. Serve immediately.

Nutrition Info:
• Per Serving: Calories: 260;Fat: 14g;Protein: 28g;Carbs: 6.5g.

Date Lamb Tangine

Servings:4
Cooking Time:40 Minutes

Ingredients:
• 2 tbsp olive oil
• 1 tbsp dates, chopped
• 1 lb lamb, cubed
• 1 garlic clove, minced
• 1 onion, grated
• 2 tbsp orange juice
• Salt and black pepper to taste
• 1 cup vegetable stock

Directions:
1. Warm the olive oil in a skillet over medium heat and cook onion and garlic for 5 minutes. Put in lamb and cook for another 5 minutes. Stir in dates, orange juice, salt, pepper, and stock and bring to a boil; cook for 20 minutes. Serve.

Nutrition Info:
• Per Serving: Calories: 298;Fat: 14g;Protein: 17g;Carbs: 19g.

Parsley Pork Stew

Servings:4
Cooking Time:8 Hours 10 Minutes

Ingredients:
• 2 tbsp olive oil
• 1 lb pork stew meat, cubed
• ½ cup chicken stock
• Salt and black pepper to taste
• 2 cups tomatoes, chopped
• 2 carrots, chopped
• 1 red bell pepper, chopped
• 1 green bell pepper, chopped
• 1 tbsp parsley, chopped

Directions:
1. Place oil, chicken stock, bell peppers, salt, pepper, pork meat, tomatoes, and carrots in your slow cooker. Cover with the lid and cook for 8 hours on Low. Scatter with parsley.

Nutrition Info:
• Per Serving: Calories: 310;Fat: 16g;Protein: 12g;Carbs: 16g.

Parsley-dijon Chicken And Potatoes

Servings:6
Cooking Time: 22 Minutes

Ingredients:
• 1 tablespoon extra-virgin olive oil
• 1½ pounds boneless, skinless chicken thighs, cut into 1-inch cubes, patted dry
• 1½ pounds Yukon Gold potatoes, unpeeled, cut into ½-inch cubes
• 2 garlic cloves, minced
• ¼ cup dry white wine
• 1 cup low-sodium or no-salt-added chicken broth
• 1 tablespoon Dijon mustard
• ¼ teaspoon freshly ground black pepper
• ¼ teaspoon kosher or sea salt
• 1 cup chopped fresh flat-leaf (Italian) parsley, including stems
• 1 tablespoon freshly squeezed lemon juice

Directions:
1. In a large skillet over medium-high heat, heat the oil. Add the chicken and cook for 5 minutes, stirring only after the chicken has browned on one side. Remove the chicken and reserve on a plate.
2. Add the potatoes to the skillet and cook for 5 minutes, stirring only after the potatoes have become golden and crispy on one side. Push the potatoes to the side of the skillet, add the garlic, and cook, stirring constantly, for 1 minute. Add the wine and cook for 1 minute, until nearly evaporated. Add the chicken broth, mustard, salt, pepper, and reserved chicken. Turn the heat to high and bring to a boil.
3. Once boiling, cover, reduce the heat to medium-low, and cook for 10 to 12 minutes, until the potatoes are tender and the internal temperature of the chicken measures 165°F on a meat thermometer and any juices run clear.
4. During the last minute of cooking, stir in the parsley. Remove from the heat, stir in the lemon juice, and serve.

Nutrition Info:
• Per Serving: Calories: 324;Fat: 9.0g;Protein: 16.0g;-Carbs: 45.0g.

Greek-style Chicken With Potatoes

Servings:4
Cooking Time:30 Minutes

Ingredients:
• 4 potatoes, peeled and quartered
• 4 boneless skinless chicken drumsticks
• 4 cups water
• 2 lemons, zested and juiced
• 1 tbsp olive oil
• 2 tsp fresh oregano

- Salt and black pepper to taste
- 2 Serrano peppers, minced
- 3 tbsp finely chopped parsley
- 1 cup packed watercress
- 1 cucumber, thinly chopped
- 10 cherry tomatoes, quartered
- 16 Kalamata olives, pitted
- ¼ cup hummus
- ¼ cup feta cheese, crumbled
- Lemon wedges, for serving

Directions:

1. Add water and potatoes to your Instant Pot. Set trivet over them. In a baking bowl, mix lemon juice, olive oil, black pepper, oregano, zest, salt, and Serrano peppers. Add chicken drumsticks in the marinade and stir to coat.

2. Set the bowl with chicken on the trivet in the cooker. Seal the lid, select Manual and cook on High for 15 minutes. Do a quick release. Take out the bowl with chicken and the trivet from the pot. Drain potatoes and add parsley and salt. Split the potatoes among serving plates and top with watercress, cucumber slices, hummus, cherry tomatoes, chicken, olives, and feta cheese. Garnish with lemon wedges. Serve.

Nutrition Info:

- Per Serving: Calories: 726;Fat: 15g;Protein: 72g;Carbs: 75g.

Chicken Drumsticks With Peach Glaze

Servings:4
Cooking Time:35 Minutes

Ingredients:

- 2 tbsp olive oil
- 8 chicken drumsticks, skinless
- 3 peaches, peeled and chopped
- ¼ cup honey
- ¼ cup cider vinegar
- 1 sweet onion, chopped
- 1 tsp minced fresh rosemary
- Salt to taste

Directions:

1. Warm the olive oil in a large skillet over medium heat. Sprinkle chicken with salt and pepper and brown it for about 7 minutes per side. Remove to a plate. Add onion and rosemary to the skillet and sauté for 1 minute or until lightly golden. Add honey, vinegar, salt, and peaches and cook for 10-12 minutes or until peaches are softened. Add the chicken back to the skillet and heat just until warm, brushing with the sauce. Serve chicken thighs with peach sauce. Enjoy!

Nutrition Info:

- Per Serving: Calories: 1492;Fat: 26g;Protein: 54g;Carbs:

27g.

Honey Mustard Pork Chops

Servings:4
Cooking Time:40 Minutes

Ingredients:

- 2 tbsp olive oil
- ½ cup vegetable stock
- 2 tbsp wholegrain mustard
- 1 tbsp honey
- 4 pork loin chops, boneless
- Salt and black pepper to taste

Directions:

1. Preheat oven to 380 F. Mix honey, mustard, salt, pepper, paprika, and olive oil in a bowl. Add in the pork and toss to coat. Transfer to a greased baking sheet and pour in the vegetable stock. Bake covered with foil for 30 minutes. Remove the foil and bake for 6-8 minutes until golden brown.

Nutrition Info:

- Per Serving: Calories: 180;Fat: 6g;Protein: 26g;Carbs: 3g.

Juicy Pork Chops

Servings:4
Cooking Time:30 Minutes

Ingredients:

- 3 tbsp olive oil
- 4 pork chops
- Salt and black pepper to taste
- 5 tbsp chicken broth
- 6 garlic cloves, minced
- ¼ cup honey
- 2 tbsp apple cider vinegar
- 2 tbsp parsley, chopped

Directions:

1. Warm the olive oil in a large skillet over medium heat. Season the pork chops with salt and pepper and add them to the skillet. Cook for 10 minutes on both sides or until golden brown; reserve. Lower the heat and add 3 tablespoons of broth, scraping the bits and flavors from the bottom of the skillet; cook for 2 minutes until the broth evaporates. Add the garlic and cook for 30 seconds. Stir in honey, vinegar, and the remaining broth. Cook for 3-4 minutes until the sauce thickens slightly. Return the pork chops and cook for 2 minutes. Top with parsley and serve.

Nutrition Info:

- Per Serving: Calories: 302;Fat: 16g;Protein: 22g;Carbs: 19g.

Marsala Chicken With Mushrooms

Servings:4
Cooking Time:30 Minutes

Ingredients:
- 4 chicken breasts, pounded thin
- ¼ cup olive oil
- Salt and black pepper to taste
- ¼ cup whole-wheat flour
- ½ lb mushrooms, sliced
- 2 carrots, chopped
- 1 cup Marsala wine
- 1 cup chicken broth
- ¼ cup parsley, chopped

Directions:
1. Warm the olive oil in a saucepan on medium heat. Season the chicken with salt and pepper, then dredge them in the flour. Fry until golden brown on both sides, about 4-6 minutes; reserve. Sauté the mushrooms and carrots in the same pan. Add the wine and chicken broth and bring to a simmer. Cook for 10 minutes or until the sauce is reduced and thickened slightly. Return the chicken to the pan, and cook it in the sauce for 10 minutes. Top with parsley and serve.

Nutrition Info:
- Per Serving: Calories: 869;Fat: 36g;Protein: 89g;Carbs: 49g.

Pork Chops In Wine Sauce

Servings:4
Cooking Time:30 Minutes

Ingredients:
- 2 tbsp olive oil
- 4 pork chops
- 1 cup red onion, sliced
- 10 black peppercorns, crushed
- ¼ cup vegetable stock
- ¼ cup dry white wine
- 2 garlic cloves, minced
- Salt to taste

Directions:
1. Warm the olive oil in a skillet over medium heat and sear pork chops for 8 minutes on both sides. Put in onion and garlic and cook for another 2 minutes. Mix in stock, wine, salt, and peppercorns and cook for 10 minutes, stirring often.

Nutrition Info:
- Per Serving: Calories: 240;Fat: 10g;Protein: 25g;Carbs: 14g.

Tomato Walnut Chicken

Servings:4
Cooking Time:35 Minutes

Ingredients:
- 2 tbsp olive oil
- 1 lb chicken breast halves
- Salt and black pepper to taste
- 2 tbsp walnuts, chopped
- 1 tbsp chives, chopped
- ½ cup tomato sauce
- ½ cup chicken stock

Directions:
1. Warm the olive oil in a skillet over medium heat and cook chicken for 8 minutes, flipping once. Season with salt and pepper. Stir in walnuts, tomato sauce, and stock and bring to a boil. Cook for 16 minutes. Serve sprinkled with chives.

Nutrition Info:
- Per Serving: Calories: 300;Fat: 13g;Protein: 36g;Carbs: 26g.

Greek-style Veggie & Beef In Pita

Servings:2
Cooking Time:30 Minutes

Ingredients:
- Beef
- 1 tbsp olive oil
- ½ medium onion, minced
- 2 garlic cloves, minced
- 6 oz lean ground beef
- 1 tsp dried oregano
- Yogurt Sauce
- ⅓ cup plain Greek yogurt
- 1 oz crumbled feta cheese
- 1 tbsp minced fresh dill
- 1 tbsp minced scallions
- 1 tbsp lemon juice
- Garlic salt to taste
- Sandwiches
- 2 Greek-style pitas, warm
- 6 cherry tomatoes, halved
- 1 cucumber, sliced
- Salt and black pepper to taste

Directions:
1. Warm the 1 tbsp olive oil in a pan over medium heat. Sauté the onion, garlic, and ground for 5-7 minutes, breaking up the meat well. When the meat is no longer pink, drain off any fat and stir in oregano. Turn off the heat.
2. In a small bowl, combine the yogurt, feta, dill, scallions, lemon juice, and garlic salt. Divide the yogurt sauce

between the warm pitas. Top with ground beef, cherry tomatoes, and diced cucumber. Season with salt and pepper. Serve.

Nutrition Info:
- Per Serving: Calories: 541;Fat: 21g;Protein: 29g;Carbs: 57g.

Herby Chicken With Asparagus Sauce

Servings:4
Cooking Time:40 Minutes

Ingredients:
- 1 chicken legs
- 4 garlic cloves, minced
- 4 fresh thyme, minced
- 3 fresh rosemary, minced
- Salt and black pepper to taste
- 2 tbsp olive oil
- 8 oz asparagus, chopped
- 1 onion, chopped
- 1 cup chicken stock
- 1 tbsp soy sauce
- 1 fresh thyme sprig
- 1 tbsp flour
- 2 tbsp parsley, chopped

Directions:
1. Warm the olive oil on Sauté in your Instant Pot. Add in onion and asparagus and sauté for 5 minutes until softened. Pour in chicken stock, 1 thyme sprig, black pepper, soy sauce, and salt, and stir. Insert a trivet over the asparagus mixture. Rub all sides of the chicken with garlic, rosemary, black pepper, lemon zest, thyme, and salt. Arrange the chicken legs on the trivet. Seal the lid, select Manual, and cook for 20 minutes on High Pressure. Do a quick release. Remove the chicken to a serving platter. In the inner pot, sprinkle flour over the asparagus mixture and blend the sauce with an immersion blender until desired consistency. Top the chicken with asparagus sauce and garnish with parsley. Serve and enjoy!

Nutrition Info:
- Per Serving: Calories: 193;Fat: 11g;Protein: 16g;Carbs: 10g.

Peach Pork Chops

Servings:4
Cooking Time:30 Minutes

Ingredients:
- 2 tbsp olive oil
- ½ tsp cayenne powder
- 4 pork chops, boneless
- ¼ cup peach preserves
- 1 tbsp thyme, chopped

Directions:
1. In a bowl, mix peach preserves, olive oil, and cayenne powder. Preheat your grill to medium. Rub pork chops with some peach glaze and grill for 10 minutes. Turn the chops, rub more glaze and cook for 10 minutes. Top with thyme.

Nutrition Info:
- Per Serving: Calories: 240;Fat: 12g;Protein: 24g;Carbs: 7g.

Garlicky Beef With Walnuts

Servings:4
Cooking Time:30 Minutes

Ingredients:
- 3 tbsp olive oil
- 1 ½ lb beef meat, cubed
- 2 tbsp lime juice
- 1 tbsp balsamic vinegar
- 5 garlic cloves, minced
- Salt and black pepper to taste
- 2 tbsp walnuts, chopped
- 2 scallions, chopped

Directions:
1. Warm the olive oil in a skillet over medium heat and sear beef for 8 minutes on both sides. Put in scallions and garlic and cook for another 2 minutes. Stir in lime juice, vinegar, salt, pepper, and walnuts and cook for an additional 10 minutes.

Nutrition Info:
- Per Serving: Calories: 310;Fat: 15g;Protein: 19g;Carbs: 17g.

Easy Pork Stew

Servings:4
Cooking Time:50 Minutes

Ingredients:
- 1 tbsp olive oil
- 1 lb pork stew meat, cubed
- 2 shallots, chopped
- 14 oz canned tomatoes, diced
- 1 garlic clove, minced
- 3 cups beef stock
- 2 tbsp paprika
- 1 tsp coriander seeds
- 1 tsp dried thyme
- Salt and black pepper to taste
- 2 tbsp parsley, chopped

Directions:
1. Warm the olive oil in a pot over medium heat and cook pork meat for 5 minutes until brown, stirring occasionally. Add in shallots and garlic and cook for an additional 3 min-

utes. Stir in beef stock, tomatoes, paprika, thyme, coriander seeds, salt, and pepper and bring to a boil; cook for 30 minutes. Serve warm topped with parsley.

Nutrition Info:
• Per Serving: Calories: 330;Fat: 18g;Protein: 35g;Carbs: 28g.

Potato Lamb And Olive Stew

Servings:10
Cooking Time: 3 Hours 42 Minutes

Ingredients:
• 4 tablespoons almond flour
• ¾ cup low-sodium chicken stock
• 1¼ pounds small potatoes, halved
• 3 cloves garlic, minced
• 4 large shallots, cut into ½-inch wedges
• 3 sprigs fresh rosemary
• 1 tablespoon lemon zest
• Coarse sea salt and black pepper, to taste
• 3½ pounds lamb shanks, fat trimmed and cut crosswise into 1½-inch pieces
• 2 tablespoons extra-virgin olive oil
• ½ cup dry white wine
• 1 cup pitted green olives, halved
• 2 tablespoons lemon juice

Directions:
1. Combine 1 tablespoon of almond flour with chicken stock in a bowl. Stir to mix well.
2. Put the flour mixture, potatoes, garlic, shallots, rosemary, and lemon zest in the slow cooker. Sprinkle with salt and black pepper. Stir to mix well. Set aside.
3. Combine the remaining almond flour with salt and black pepper in a large bowl, then dunk the lamb shanks in the flour and toss to coat.
4. Heat the olive oil in a nonstick skillet over medium-high heat until shimmering.
5. Add the well-coated lamb and cook for 10 minutes or until golden brown. Flip the lamb pieces halfway through the cooking time. Transfer the cooked lamb to the slow cooker.
6. Pour the wine in the same skillet, then cook for 2 minutes or until it reduces in half. Pour the wine in the slow cooker.
7. Put the slow cooker lid on and cook on high for 3 hours and 30 minutes or until the lamb is very tender.
8. In the last 20 minutes of the cooking, open the lid and fold in the olive halves to cook.
9. Pour the stew on a large plate, let them sit for 5 minutes, then skim any fat remains over the face of the liquid.
10. Drizzle with lemon juice and sprinkle with salt and pepper. Serve warm.

Nutrition Info:

• Per Serving: Calories: 309;Fat: 10.3g;Protein: 36.9g;Carbs: 16.1g.

French Chicken Cassoulet

Servings:4
Cooking Time:40 Minutes

Ingredients:
• 1 tbsp olive oil
• ½ cup heavy cream
• 4 chicken breasts, halved
• 1/3 cup yellow mustard
• Salt and black pepper to taste
• 1 onion, chopped
• 1 ½ cups chicken stock
• ¼ tsp dried oregano

Directions:
1. Warm stock in a saucepan over medium heat and stir in mustard, onion, salt, pepper, and oregano. Bring to a boil and cook for 8 minutes. Warm olive oil in a skillet over medium heat. Sear chicken for 6 minutes on both sides. Transfer to the saucepan and simmer for another 12 minutes. Stir in heavy cream for 2 minutes. Serve warm.

Nutrition Info:
• Per Serving: Calories: 260;Fat: 12g;Protein: 27g;Carbs: 18g.

Greek-style Lamb Burgers

Servings:4
Cooking Time: 10 Minutes

Ingredients:
• 1 pound ground lamb
• ½ teaspoon salt
• ½ teaspoon freshly ground black pepper
• 4 tablespoons crumbled feta cheese
• Buns, toppings, and tzatziki, for serving (optional)

Directions:
1. Preheat the grill to high heat.
2. In a large bowl, using your hands, combine the lamb with the salt and pepper.
3. Divide the meat into 4 portions. Divide each portion in half to make a top and a bottom. Flatten each half into a 3-inch circle. Make a dent in the center of one of the halves and place 1 tablespoon of the feta cheese in the center. Place the second half of the patty on top of the feta cheese and press down to close the 2 halves together, making it resemble a round burger.
4. Grill each side for 3 minutes, for medium-well. Serve on a bun with your favorite toppings and tzatziki sauce, if desired.

Nutrition Info:

• Per Serving: Calories: 345;Fat: 29.0g;Protein: 20.0g;-Carbs: 1.0g.

Beef Cherry & Tomato Cassoulet

Servings:4
Cooking Time:30 Minutes

Ingredients:
• 3 tbsp olive oil
• 2 garlic cloves, minced
• 1 lemon, juiced and zested
• 1 ½ lb ground beef
• Salt and black pepper to taste
• 1 lb cherry tomatoes, halved
• 1 red onion, chopped
• 2 tbsp tomato paste
• 1 tbsp mint leaves, chopped

Directions:
1. Warm the olive oil in a skillet over medium heat and cook beef and garlic for 5 minutes. Stir in lemon zest, lemon juice, salt, pepper, cherry tomatoes, onion, tomato paste, and mint and cook for 15 minutes. Serve right away.

Nutrition Info:
• Per Serving: Calories: 324;Fat: 10g;Protein: 16g;Carbs: 22g.

Citrus Chicken Wings

Servings:6
Cooking Time:50 Minutes

Ingredients:
• 2 tbsp canola oils
• 12 chicken wings, halved
• 2 garlic cloves, minced
• 1 lime, juiced and zested
• 1 cup raisins, soaked
• 1 tsp cumin, ground
• Salt and black pepper to taste
• ½ cup chicken stock
• 1 tbsp chives, chopped

Directions:
1. Preheat the oven to 340 F. Combine chicken wings, garlic, lime juice, lime zest, canola oil, raisins, cumin, salt, pepper, stock, and chives in a baking pan. Bake for 40 minutes.

Nutrition Info:
• Per Serving: Calories: 300;Fat: 20g;Protein: 19g;Carbs: 22g.

Grilled Lemon Chicken

Servings:2
Cooking Time: 12 To 14 Minutes

Ingredients:
• Marinade:
• 4 tablespoons freshly squeezed lemon juice
• 2 tablespoons olive oil, plus more for greasing the grill grates
• 1 teaspoon dried basil
• 1 teaspoon paprika
• ½ teaspoon dried thyme
• ¼ teaspoon salt
• ¼ teaspoon garlic powder
• 2 boneless, skinless chicken breasts

Directions:
1. Make the marinade: Whisk together the lemon juice, olive oil, basil, paprika, thyme, salt, and garlic powder in a large bowl until well combined.
2. Add the chicken breasts to the bowl and let marinate for at least 30 minutes.
3. When ready to cook, preheat the grill to medium-high heat. Lightly grease the grill grates with the olive oil.
4. Discard the marinade and arrange the chicken breasts on the grill grates.
5. Grill for 12 to 14 minutes, flipping the chicken halfway through, or until a meat thermometer inserted in the center of the chicken reaches 165ºF.
6. Let the chicken cool for 5 minutes and serve warm.

Nutrition Info:
• Per Serving: Calories: 251;Fat: 15.5g;Protein: 27.3g;-Carbs: 1.9g.

Rosemary Spatchcock Chicken

Servings:6
Cooking Time:55 Minutes

Ingredients:
• 2 tbsp butter, melted
• 2 tbsp olive oil
• 1 whole chicken
• 8 garlic cloves, chopped
• 2 tbsp rosemary, chopped
• Salt and black pepper to taste
• 2 lemons, thinly sliced

Directions:
1. Preheat oven to 425 F. Put the chicken breast side down on a work surface. With a sharp knife, cut along the backbone, starting at the tail end and working your way up to the neck. Pull apart the two sides, opening up the chicken. Turn it over, breast-side up, pressing down with your hands to flatten the bird. Transfer to a greased baking dish. Loosen

the skin over the breasts and thighs by cutting a small incision and sticking one or two fingers inside to pull the skin away from the meat without removing it.

2. In a small bowl, whisk the olive oil, garlic, rosemary, salt, and pepper. Rub the mixture under the skin of each breast and each thigh. Add the lemon slices evenly to the same areas. Mix the melted butter, salt, and pepper and rub over the outside of the chicken. Roast the chicken for 40-45 minutes or until cooked through, and the skin is golden and charred. Leave to rest for 10 minutes, then slice to serve.

Nutrition Info:
• Per Serving: Calories: 435;Fat: 34g;Protein: 28g;Carbs: 2g.

Mustardy Steak In Mushroom Sauce

Servings:4
Cooking Time:30 Min + Marinating Time

Ingredients:
• For the steak
• 2 tbsp olive oil
• 1 lb beef skirt steak
• 1 cup red wine
• 2 garlic cloves, minced
• 1 tbsp Worcestershire sauce
• 1 tbsp dried thyme
• 1 tsp yellow mustard
• For the mushroom sauce
• 1 lb mushrooms, sliced
• 1 tsp dried dill
• 2 garlic cloves, minced
• 1 cup dry red wine
• Salt and black pepper to taste

Directions:
1. Combine wine, garlic, Worcestershire sauce, 2 tbsp of olive oil, thyme, and mustard in a bowl. Place in the steak, cover with plastic wrap and let it marinate for at least 3 hours in the refrigerator. Remove the steak and pat dry with paper towels.

2. Warm olive oil in a pan over medium heat and sear steak for 8 minutes on all sides; set aside. In the same pan, sauté mushrooms, dill, salt, and pepper for 6 minutes, stirring periodically. Add in garlic and sauté for 30 seconds. Pour in the wine and scrape off any bits from the bottom. Simmer for 5 minutes until the liquid reduces. Slice the steak and top with the mushroom sauce. Serve hot.

Nutrition Info:
• Per Serving: Calories: 424;Fat: 24g;Protein: 29g;Carbs: 8g.

Shallot Beef

Servings:4
Cooking Time:50 Minutes

Ingredients:
• 2 tbsp olive oil
• 1 lb beef meat, cubed
• 1 lb shallots, chopped
• 1 tbsp sweet paprika
• Salt and black pepper to taste
• 1 ½ cups chicken stock
• 4 garlic cloves, minced
• 1 cup balsamic vinegar

Directions:
1. Warm the olive oil in a pot over medium heat and sauté shallots, balsamic vinegar, salt, and pepper for 10 minutes. Stir in beef, paprika, chicken stock, and garlic and bring to a simmer. Cook for 30 minutes. Serve immediately.

Nutrition Info:
• Per Serving: Calories: 312;Fat: 13g;Protein: 18g;Carbs: 16g.

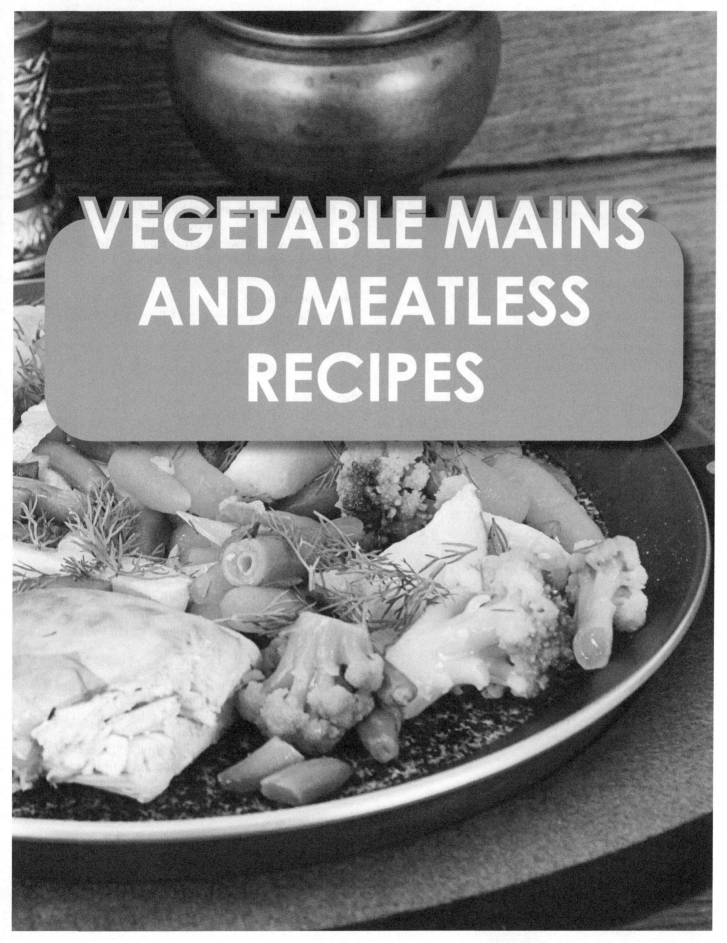

VEGETABLE MAINS AND MEATLESS RECIPES

Authentic Mushroom Gratin

Servings:4
Cooking Time:25 Minutes

Ingredients:
- 2 lb Button mushrooms, cleaned
- 2 tbsp olive oil
- 2 tomatoes, sliced
- 2 tomato paste
- ½ cup Parmesan cheese, grated
- ½ cup dry white wine
- ¼ tsp sweet paprika
- ½ tsp dried basil
- ½ tsp dried thyme
- Salt and black pepper to taste

Directions:
1. Preheat oven to 360 F. Combine tomatoes, tomato paste, wine, oil, mushrooms, paprika, black pepper, salt, basil, and thyme in a baking dish. Bake for 15 minutes. Top with Parmesan and continue baking for 5 minutes until the cheese melts.

Nutrition Info:
- Per Serving: Calories: 162;Fat: 8.6g;Protein: 9g;Carbs: 12.3g.

Braised Cauliflower With White Wine

Servings:4
Cooking Time: 12 To 16 Minutes

Ingredients:
- 3 tablespoons plus 1 teaspoon extra-virgin olive oil, divided
- 3 garlic cloves, minced
- ⅛ teaspoon red pepper flakes
- 1 head cauliflower, cored and cut into 1½-inch florets
- ¼ teaspoon salt, plus more for seasoning
- Black pepper, to taste
- ⅓ cup vegetable broth
- ⅓ cup dry white wine
- 2 tablespoons minced fresh parsley

Directions:
1. Combine 1 teaspoon of the oil, garlic and pepper flakes in small bowl.
2. Heat the remaining 3 tablespoons of the oil in a skillet over medium-high heat until shimmering. Add the cauliflower and ¼ teaspoon of the salt and cook for 7 to 9 minutes, stirring occasionally, or until florets are golden brown.
3. Push the cauliflower to sides of the skillet. Add the garlic mixture to the center of the skillet. Cook for about 30 seconds, or until fragrant. Stir the garlic mixture into the cauliflower.
4. Pour in the broth and wine and bring to simmer. Reduce the heat to medium-low. Cover and cook for 4 to 6 minutes, or until the cauliflower is crisp-tender. Off heat, stir in the parsley and season with salt and pepper.
5. Serve immediately.

Nutrition Info:
- Per Serving: Calories: 143;Fat: 11.7g;Protein: 3.1g;-Carbs: 8.7g.

Garlicky Broccoli Rabe

Servings:4
Cooking Time: 5 To 6 Minutes

Ingredients:
- 14 ounces broccoli rabe, trimmed and cut into 1-inch pieces
- 2 teaspoons salt, plus more for seasoning
- Black pepper, to taste
- 2 tablespoons extra-virgin olive oil
- 3 garlic cloves, minced
- ¼ teaspoon red pepper flakes

Directions:
1. Bring 3 quarts water to a boil in a large saucepan. Add the broccoli rabe and 2 teaspoons of the salt to the boiling water and cook for 2 to 3 minutes, or until wilted and tender.
2. Drain the broccoli rabe. Transfer to ice water and let sit until chilled. Drain again and pat dry.
3. In a skillet over medium heat, heat the oil and add the garlic and red pepper flakes. Sauté for about 2 minutes, or until the garlic begins to sizzle.
4. Increase the heat to medium-high. Stir in the broccoli rabe and cook for about 1 minute, or until heated through, stirring constantly. Season with salt and pepper.
5. Serve immediately.

Nutrition Info:
- Per Serving: Calories: 87;Fat: 7.3g;Protein: 3.4g;Carbs: 4.0g.

Balsamic Grilled Vegetables

Servings:4
Cooking Time:20 Minutes

Ingredients:
- ¼ cup olive oil
- 4 carrots, cut in half
- 2 onions, quartered
- 1 zucchini, cut into rounds
- 1 eggplant, cut into rounds
- 1 red bell pepper, chopped
- Salt and black pepper to taste
- Balsamic vinegar to taste

Directions:
1. Heat your grill to medium-high. Brush the vegetables lightly with olive oil, and season with salt and pepper. Grill the vegetables for 3–4 minutes per side. Transfer to a serving dish and drizzle with balsamic vinegar. Serve and enjoy!

Nutrition Info:
- Per Serving: Calories: 184;Fat: 14g;Protein: 2.1g;Carbs: 14g.

Parmesan Asparagus With Tomatoes

Servings:6
Cooking Time:30 Minutes

Ingredients:
- 3 tbsp olive oil
- 2 garlic cloves, minced
- 12 oz cherry tomatoes, halved
- 1 tsp dried oregano
- 10 Kalamata olives, chopped
- 2 lb asparagus, trimmed
- 2 tbsp fresh basil, chopped
- ¼ cup Parmesan cheese, grated
- Salt and black pepper to taste

Directions:
1. Warm 2 tbsp of olive oil in a skillet over medium heat sauté the garlic for 1-2 minutes, stirring often, until golden. Add tomatoes, olives, and oregano and cook until tomatoes begin to break down, about 3 minutes; transfer to a bowl.
2. Coat the asparagus with the remaining olive oil and cook in a grill pan over medium heat for about 5 minutes, turning once until crisp-tender. Sprinkle with salt and pepper. Transfer asparagus to a serving platter, top with tomato mixture, and sprinkle with basil and Parmesan cheese. Serve and enjoy!

Nutrition Info:
- Per Serving: Calories: 157;Fat: 7g;Protein: 7.3g;Carbs: 19g.

Sautéed Cabbage With Parsley

Servings:4
Cooking Time: 12 To 14 Minutes

Ingredients:
- 1 small head green cabbage, cored and sliced thin
- 2 tablespoons extra-virgin olive oil, divided
- 1 onion, halved and sliced thin
- ¾ teaspoon salt, divided
- ¼ teaspoon black pepper
- ¼ cup chopped fresh parsley
- 1½ teaspoons lemon juice

Directions:
1. Place the cabbage in a large bowl with cold water. Let sit for 3 minutes. Drain well.
2. Heat 1 tablespoon of the oil in a skillet over medium-high heat until shimmering. Add the onion and ¼ teaspoon of the salt and cook for 5 to 7 minutes, or until softened and lightly browned. Transfer to a bowl.
3. Heat the remaining 1 tablespoon of the oil in now-empty skillet over medium-high heat until shimmering. Add the cabbage and sprinkle with the remaining ½ teaspoon of the salt and black pepper. Cover and cook for about 3 minutes, without stirring, or until cabbage is wilted and lightly browned on bottom.
4. Stir and continue to cook for about 4 minutes, uncovered, or until the cabbage is crisp-tender and lightly browned in places, stirring once halfway through cooking. Off heat, stir in the cooked onion, parsley and lemon juice.
5. Transfer to a plate and serve.

Nutrition Info:
- Per Serving: Calories: 117;Fat: 7.0g;Protein: 2.7g;Carbs: 13.4g.

Simple Oven-baked Green Beans

Servings:6
Cooking Time:15 Minutes

Ingredients:
- 2 tbsp olive oil
- 2 lb green beans, trimmed
- Salt and black pepper to taste

Directions:
1. Preheat oven to 400 F. Toss the green beans with some olive oil, salt, and spread them in a single layer on a greased baking dish. Roast for 8-10 minutes. Transfer green beans to a serving platter and drizzle with the remaining olive oil.

Nutrition Info:
- Per Serving: Calories: 157;Fat: 2g;Protein: 3g;Carbs: 6g.

Tradicional Matchuba Green Beans

Servings:4
Cooking Time:15 Minutes

Ingredients:
- 1 ¼ lb narrow green beans, trimmed
- 3 tbsp butter, melted
- 1 cup Moroccan matbucha
- 2 green onions, chopped
- Salt and black pepper to taste

Directions:
1. Steam the green beans in a pot for 5-6 minutes until tender. Remove to a bowl, reserving the cooking liquid. In a skillet over medium heat, melt the butter. Add in green onions, salt, and black pepper and cook until fragrant. Lower the heat and put in the green beans along with some of the reserved water. Simmer for 3-4 minutes. Serve the green beans with the Sabra Moroccan matbucha as a dip.

Nutrition Info:
- Per Serving: Calories: 125;Fat: 8.6g;Protein: 2.2g;Carbs: 9g.

Baked Vegetable Stew

Servings:6
Cooking Time:70 Minutes

Ingredients:
- 1 can diced tomatoes, drained with juice reserved
- 3 tbsp olive oil
- 1 onion, chopped
- 2 tbsp fresh oregano, minced
- 1 tsp paprika
- 4 garlic cloves, minced
- 1 ½ lb green beans, sliced
- 1 lb Yukon Gold potatoes, peeled and chopped
- 1 tbsp tomato paste
- Salt and black pepper to taste
- 3 tbsp fresh basil, chopped

Directions:
1. Preheat oven to 360 F. Warm the olive oil in a skillet over medium heat. Sauté onion and garlic for 3 minutes until softened. Stir in oregano and paprika for 30 seconds. Transfer to a baking dish and add in green beans, potatoes, tomatoes, tomato paste, salt, pepper, and 1 ½ cups of water; stir well. Bake for 40-50 minutes. Sprinkle with basil. Serve.

Nutrition Info:
- Per Serving: Calories: 121;Fat: 0.8g;Protein: 4.2g;Carbs: 26g.

Zoodles With Walnut Pesto

Servings:4
Cooking Time: 10 Minutes

Ingredients:
- 4 medium zucchinis, spiralized
- ¼ cup extra-virgin olive oil, divided
- 1 teaspoon minced garlic, divided
- ½ teaspoon crushed red pepper
- ¼ teaspoon freshly ground black pepper, divided
- ¼ teaspoon kosher salt, divided
- 2 tablespoons grated Parmesan cheese, divided
- 1 cup packed fresh basil leaves
- ¾ cup walnut pieces, divided

Directions:
1. In a large bowl, stir together the zoodles, 1 tablespoon of the olive oil, ½ teaspoon of the minced garlic, red pepper, ⅛ teaspoon of the black pepper and ⅛ teaspoon of the salt. Set aside.
2. Heat ½ tablespoon of the oil in a large skillet over medium-high heat. Add half of the zoodles to the skillet and cook for 5 minutes, stirring constantly. Transfer the cooked zoodles into a bowl. Repeat with another ½ tablespoon of the oil and the remaining zoodles. When done, add the cooked zoodles to the bowl.
3. Make the pesto: In a food processor, combine the remaining ½ teaspoon of the minced garlic, ⅛ teaspoon of the black pepper and ⅛ teaspoon of the salt, 1 tablespoon of the Parmesan, basil leaves and ¼ cup of the walnuts. Pulse until smooth and then slowly drizzle the remaining 2 tablespoons of the oil into the pesto. Pulse again until well combined.
4. Add the pesto to the zoodles along with the remaining 1 tablespoon of the Parmesan and the remaining ½ cup of the walnuts. Toss to coat well.
5. Serve immediately.

Nutrition Info:
- Per Serving: Calories: 166;Fat: 16.0g;Protein: 4.0g;-Carbs: 3.0g.

Easy Zucchini Patties

Servings:2
Cooking Time: 5 Minutes

Ingredients:
- 2 medium zucchinis, shredded
- 1 teaspoon salt, divided
- 2 eggs
- 2 tablespoons chickpea flour
- 1 tablespoon chopped fresh mint
- 1 scallion, chopped
- 2 tablespoons extra-virgin olive oil

Directions:
1. Put the shredded zucchini in a fine-mesh strainer and season with ½ teaspoon of salt. Set aside.
2. Beat together the eggs, chickpea flour, mint, scallion, and remaining ½ teaspoon of salt in a medium bowl.
3. Squeeze the zucchini to drain as much liquid as possible. Add the zucchini to the egg mixture and stir until well incorporated.
4. Heat the olive oil in a large skillet over medium-high heat.
5. Drop the zucchini mixture by spoonful into the skillet. Gently flatten the zucchini with the back of a spatula.
6. Cook for 2 to 3 minutes or until golden brown. Flip and cook for an additional 2 minutes.
7. Remove from the heat and serve on a plate.

Nutrition Info:
- Per Serving: Calories: 264;Fat: 20.0g;Protein: 9.8g;- Carbs: 16.1g.

Roasted Celery Root With Yogurt Sauce

Servings:6
Cooking Time:50 Minutes

Ingredients:
- 3 tbsp olive oil
- 3 celery roots, sliced
- Salt and black pepper to taste
- ¼ cup plain yogurt
- ¼ tsp grated lemon zest
- 1 tsp lemon juice
- 1 tsp sesame seeds, toasted
- 1 tsp coriander seeds, crushed
- ¼ tsp dried thyme
- ¼ tsp chili powder
- ¼ cup fresh cilantro, chopped

Directions:
1. Preheat oven to 425 F. Place the celery slices on a baking sheet. Sprinkle them with olive oil, salt, and pepper. Roast for 25-30 minutes. Flip each piece and continue to roast for 10-15 minutes until celery root is very tender and sides touching sheet are browned. Transfer celery to a serving platter.
2. Whisk yogurt, lemon zest and juice, and salt together in a bowl. In a separate bowl, combine sesame seeds, coriander seeds, thyme, chili powder, and salt. Drizzle celery root with yogurt sauce and sprinkle with seed mixture and cilantro.

Nutrition Info:
- Per Serving: Calories: 75;Fat: 7.5g;Protein: 0.7g;Carbs: 1.8g.

Chargrilled Vegetable Kebabs

Servings:4
Cooking Time:26 Minutes

Ingredients:
- 2 red bell peppers, cut into squares
- 2 zucchinis, sliced into half-moons
- 6 portobello mushroom caps, quartered
- ¼ cup olive oil
- 1 tsp Dijon mustard
- 1 tsp fresh rosemary, chopped
- 1 garlic clove, minced
- Salt and black pepper to taste
- 2 red onions, cut into wedges

Directions:
1. Preheat your grill to High. Mix the olive oil, mustard, rosemary, garlic, salt, and pepper in a bowl. Reserve half of the oil mixture for serving. Thread the vegetables in alternating order onto metal skewers and brush them with the remaining oil mixture. Grill them for about 15 minutes until browned, turning occasionally. Transfer the kebabs to a serving platter and remove the skewers. Drizzle with reserved oil mixture and serve.

Nutrition Info:
- Per Serving: Calories: 96;Fat: 9.2g;Protein: 1.1g;Carbs: 3.6g.

Parmesan Stuffed Zucchini Boats

Servings:4
Cooking Time: 15 Minutes

Ingredients:
- 1 cup canned low-sodium chickpeas, drained and rinsed
- 1 cup no-sugar-added spaghetti sauce
- 2 zucchinis
- ¼ cup shredded Parmesan cheese

Directions:
1. Preheat the oven to 425ºF.
2. In a medium bowl, stir together the chickpeas and spaghetti sauce.
3. Cut the zucchini in half lengthwise and scrape a spoon gently down the length of each half to remove the seeds.
4. Fill each zucchini half with the chickpea sauce and top with one-quarter of the Parmesan cheese.
5. Place the zucchini halves on a baking sheet and roast in the oven for 15 minutes.
6. Transfer to a plate. Let rest for 5 minutes before serving.

Nutrition Info:
- Per Serving: Calories: 139;Fat: 4.0g;Protein: 8.0g;Carbs: 20.0g.

Veggie Rice Bowls With Pesto Sauce

Servings:2
Cooking Time: 1 Minute

Ingredients:
- 2 cups water
- 1 cup arborio rice, rinsed
- Salt and ground black pepper, to taste
- 2 eggs
- 1 cup broccoli florets
- ½ pound Brussels sprouts
- 1 carrot, peeled and chopped
- 1 small beet, peeled and cubed
- ¼ cup pesto sauce
- Lemon wedges, for serving

Directions:
1. Combine the water, rice, salt, and pepper in the Instant Pot. Insert a trivet over rice and place a steamer basket on top. Add the eggs, broccoli, Brussels sprouts, carrots, beet cubes, salt, and pepper to the steamer basket.
2. Lock the lid. Select the Manual mode and set the cooking time for 1 minute at High Pressure.
3. When the timer beeps, perform a natural pressure release for 10 minutes, then release any remaining pressure. Carefully open the lid.
4. Remove the steamer basket and trivet from the pot and transfer the eggs to a bowl of ice water. Peel and halve the eggs. Use a fork to fluff the rice.
5. Divide the rice, broccoli, Brussels sprouts, carrot, beet cubes, and eggs into two bowls. Top with a dollop of pesto sauce and serve with the lemon wedges.

Nutrition Info:
- Per Serving: Calories: 590;Fat: 34.1g;Protein: 21.9g; Carbs: 50.0g.

Rainbow Vegetable Kebabs

Servings:4
Cooking Time:30 Minutes

Ingredients:
- 1 cup mushrooms, cut into quarters
- 6 mixed bell peppers, cut into squares
- 4 red onions, cut into 6 wedges
- 4 zucchini, cut into half-moons
- 2 tomatoes, cut into quarters
- 3 tbsp herbed oil

Directions:
1. Preheat your grill to medium-high. Alternate the vegetables onto bamboo skewers. Grill them for 5 minutes on each side until the vegetables begin to char. Remove them from heat and drizzle with herbed oil.

Nutrition Info:
- Per Serving: Calories: 238;Fat: 12g;Protein: 6g;Carbs: 34.2g.

Chickpea Lettuce Wraps With Celery

Servings:4
Cooking Time: 0 Minutes

Ingredients:
- 1 can low-sodium chickpeas, drained and rinsed
- 1 celery stalk, thinly sliced
- 2 tablespoons finely chopped red onion
- 2 tablespoons unsalted tahini
- 3 tablespoons honey mustard
- 1 tablespoon capers, undrained
- 12 butter lettuce leaves

Directions:
1. In a bowl, mash the chickpeas with a potato masher or the back of a fork until mostly smooth.
2. Add the celery, red onion, tahini, honey mustard, and capers to the bowl and stir until well incorporated.
3. For each serving, place three overlapping lettuce leaves on a plate and top with ¼ of the mashed chickpea filling, then roll up. Repeat with the remaining lettuce leaves and chickpea mixture.

Nutrition Info:
- Per Serving: Calories: 182;Fat: 7.1g;Protein: 10.3g; Carbs: 19.6g.

Grilled Vegetable Skewers

Servings:4
Cooking Time: 10 Minutes

Ingredients:
- 4 medium red onions, peeled and sliced into 6 wedges
- 4 medium zucchini, cut into 1-inch-thick slices
- 2 beefsteak tomatoes, cut into quarters
- 4 red bell peppers, cut into 2-inch squares
- 2 orange bell peppers, cut into 2-inch squares
- 2 yellow bell peppers, cut into 2-inch squares
- 2 tablespoons plus 1 teaspoon olive oil, divided
- SPECIAL EQUIPMENT:
- 4 wooden skewers, soaked in water for at least 30 minutes

Directions:
1. Preheat the grill to medium-high heat.
2. Skewer the vegetables by alternating between red onion, zucchini, tomatoes, and the different colored bell peppers. Brush them with 2 tablespoons of olive oil.
3. Oil the grill grates with 1 teaspoon of olive oil and grill the vegetable skewers for 5 minutes. Flip the skewers and grill for 5 minutes more, or until they are cooked to your liking.
4. Let the skewers cool for 5 minutes before serving.

Nutrition Info:
- Per Serving: Calories: 115;Fat: 3.0g;Protein: 3.5g;Carbs: 18.7g.

Simple Honey-glazed Baby Carrots

Servings:2
Cooking Time: 6 Minutes

Ingredients:
- ⅔ cup water
- 1½ pounds baby carrots
- 4 tablespoons almond butter
- ½ cup honey
- 1 teaspoon dried thyme
- 1½ teaspoons dried dill
- Salt, to taste

Directions:
1. Pour the water into the Instant Pot and add a steamer basket. Place the baby carrots in the basket.
2. Secure the lid. Select the Manual mode and set the cooking time for 4 minutes at High Pressure.
3. Once cooking is complete, do a quick pressure release. Carefully open the lid.
4. Transfer the carrots to a plate and set aside.
5. Pour the water out of the Instant Pot and dry it.
6. Press the Sauté button on the Instant Pot and heat the almond butter.

7. Stir in the honey, thyme, and dill.
8. Return the carrots to the Instant Pot and stir until well coated. Sauté for another 1 minute.
9. Taste and season with salt as needed. Serve warm.

Nutrition Info:
- Per Serving: Calories: 575;Fat: 23.5g;Protein: 2.8g;Carbs: 90.6g.

Stir-fried Eggplant

Servings:2
Cooking Time: 15 Minutes

Ingredients:
- 1 cup water, plus more as needed
- ½ cup chopped red onion
- 1 tablespoon finely chopped garlic
- 1 tablespoon dried Italian herb seasoning
- 1 teaspoon ground cumin
- 1 small eggplant, peeled and cut into ½-inch cubes
- 1 medium carrot, sliced
- 2 cups green beans, cut into 1-inch pieces
- 2 ribs celery, sliced
- 1 cup corn kernels
- 2 tablespoons almond butter
- 2 medium tomatoes, chopped

Directions:
1. Heat 1 tablespoon of water in a large soup pot over medium-high heat until it sputters.
2. Cook the onion for 2 minutes, adding a little more water as needed.
3. Add the garlic, Italian seasoning, cumin, and eggplant and stir-fry for 2 to 3 minutes, adding a little more water as needed.
4. Add the carrot, green beans, celery, corn kernels, and ½ cup of water and stir well. Reduce the heat to medium, cover, and cook for 8 to 10 minutes, stirring occasionally, or until the vegetables are tender.
5. Meanwhile, in a bowl, stir together the almond butter and ½ cup of water.
6. Remove the vegetables from the heat and stir in the almond butter mixture and chopped tomatoes. Cool for a few minutes before serving.

Nutrition Info:
- Per Serving: Calories: 176;Fat: 5.5g;Protein: 5.8g;Carbs: 25.4g.

Spanish-style Green Beans With Pine Nuts

Servings:6
Cooking Time:30 Minutes

Ingredients:
- ¼ cup Manchego cheese, shredded
- ¼ cup olive oil
- 2 lb green beans, trimmed
- Salt and black pepper to taste
- 2 garlic cloves, minced
- 1 tsp Dijon mustard
- 2 tbsp fresh parsley, chopped
- 2 tbsp pine nuts, toasted

Directions:
1. Preheat oven to 420 F. Toss green beans with some olive oil, salt, and pepper. Transfer to a baking sheet and roast for 15-18 minutes, shaking occasionally the sheet. Transfer green beans to a serving plate. Microwave mixed garlic, lemon zest, salt, pepper, and the remaining olive oil for about 1 minute until bubbling. Let the mixture sit for 1 minute, then whisk in lemon juice, mustard, salt, and pepper. Drizzle the green beans with the dressing and sprinkle with basil. Top with cheese and pine nuts. Serve and enjoy!

Nutrition Info:
- Per Serving: Calories: 126;Fat: 11g;Protein: 2.6g;Carbs: 6.3g.

Roasted Asparagus With Hazelnuts

Servings:4
Cooking Time:25 Minutes

Ingredients:
- 2 tbsp olive oil
- 1 lb asparagus, trimmed
- ¼ cup hazelnuts, chopped
- 1 lemon, juiced and zested
- Salt and black pepper to taste
- ½ tsp red pepper flakes

Directions:
1. Preheat oven to 425 F. Arrange the asparagus on a baking sheet. Combine olive oil, lemon zest, lemon juice, salt, hazelnuts, and black pepper in a bowl and mix well. Pour the mixture over the asparagus. Place in the oven and roast for 15-20 minutes until tender and lightly charred. Serve topped with red pepper flakes.

Nutrition Info:
- Per Serving: Calories: 112;Fat: 10g;Protein: 3.2g;Carbs: 5.2g.

Quick Steamed Broccoli

Servings:2
Cooking Time: 0 Minutes

Ingredients:
- ¼ cup water
- 3 cups broccoli florets
- Salt and ground black pepper, to taste

Directions:
1. Pour the water into the Instant Pot and insert a steamer basket. Place the broccoli florets in the basket.
2. Secure the lid. Select the Manual mode and set the cooking time for 0 minutes at High Pressure.
3. Once cooking is complete, do a quick pressure release. Carefully open the lid.
4. Transfer the broccoli florets to a bowl with cold water to keep bright green color.
5. Season the broccoli with salt and pepper to taste, then serve.

Nutrition Info:
- Per Serving: Calories: 16;Fat: 0.2g;Protein: 1.9g;Carbs: 1.7g.

Spicy Kale With Almonds

Servings:4
Cooking Time:25 Minutes

Ingredients:
- 2 tbsp olive oil
- ¼ cup slivered almonds
- 1 lb chopped kale
- ¼ cup vegetable broth
- 1 lemon, juiced and zested
- 1 garlic clove, minced
- 1 tbsp red pepper flakes
- Salt and black pepper to taste

Directions:
1. Warm olive oil in a pan over medium heat and sauté garlic, kale, salt, and pepper for 8-9 minutes until soft. Add in lemon juice, lemon zest, red pepper flakes, and vegetable broth and continue cooking until the liquid evaporates, about 3-5 minutes. Garnish with almonds and serve.

Nutrition Info:
- Per Serving: Calories: 123;Fat: 8.1g;Protein: 4g;Carbs: 10.8g.

Hot Turnip Chickpeas

Servings:4
Cooking Time:50 Minutes

Ingredients:
- 2 tbsp olive oil
- 2 onions, chopped
- 2 red bell peppers, chopped
- Salt and black pepper to taste
- ¼ cup tomato paste
- 1 jalapeño pepper, minced
- 5 garlic cloves, minced
- ¾ tsp ground cumin
- ¼ tsp cayenne pepper
- 2 cans chickpeas
- 12 oz potatoes, chopped
- ¼ cup chopped fresh parsley
- 1 lemon, juiced

Directions:
1. Warm the olive oil in a saucepan oven over medium heat. Sauté the onions, bell peppers, salt, and pepper for 6 minutes until softened and lightly browned. Stir in tomato paste, jalapeño pepper, garlic, cumin, and cayenne pepper and cook for about 30 seconds until fragrant. Stir in chickpeas and their liquid, potatoes, and 1 cup of water. Bring to simmer and cook for 25-35 minutes until potatoes are tender and the sauce has thickened. Stir in parsley and lemon juice.

Nutrition Info:
- Per Serving: Calories: 124;Fat: 5.3g;Protein: 3.7g;Carbs: 17g.

Roasted Artichokes

Servings:4
Cooking Time:50 Minutes

Ingredients:
- 4 artichokes, stalk trimmed and large leaves removed
- 2 lemons, freshly squeezed
- 4 tbsp extra-virgin olive oil
- 4 cloves garlic, chopped
- 1 tsp fresh rosemary
- 1 tsp fresh basil
- 1 tsp fresh parsley
- 1 tsp fresh oregano
- Salt and black pepper to taste
- 1 tsp red pepper flakes
- 1 tsp paprika

Directions:
1. Preheat oven to 395 F. In a small bowl, thoroughly combine the garlic with herbs and spices; set aside. Cut the artichokes in half vertically and scoop out the fibrous choke to expose the heart with a teaspoon.
2. Rub the lemon juice all over the entire surface of the artichoke halves. Arrange them on a parchment-lined baking dish, cut side up, and brush them evenly with olive oil. Stuff the cavities with the garlic/herb mixture. Cover them with aluminum foil and bake for 30 minutes. Discard the foil and bake for another 10 minutes until lightly charred. Serve.

Nutrition Info:
- Per Serving: Calories: 220;Fat: 14g;Protein: 6g;Carbs: 21g.

Roasted Vegetables

Servings:2
Cooking Time: 35 Minutes

Ingredients:
- 6 teaspoons extra-virgin olive oil, divided
- 12 to 15 Brussels sprouts, halved
- 1 medium sweet potato, peeled and cut into 2-inch cubes
- 2 cups fresh cauliflower florets
- 1 medium zucchini, cut into 1-inch rounds
- 1 red bell pepper, cut into 1-inch slices
- Salt, to taste

Directions:
1. Preheat the oven to 425ºF.
2. Add 2 teaspoons of olive oil, Brussels sprouts, sweet potato, and salt to a large bowl and toss until they are completely coated.
3. Transfer them to a large roasting pan and roast for 10 minutes, or until the Brussels sprouts are lightly browned.
4. Meantime, combine the cauliflower florets with 2 teaspoons of olive oil and salt in a separate bowl.
5. Remove from the oven. Add the cauliflower florets to the roasting pan and roast for 10 minutes more.
6. Meanwhile, toss the zucchini and bell pepper with the remaining olive oil in a medium bowl until well coated. Season with salt.
7. Remove the roasting pan from the oven and stir in the zucchini and bell pepper. Continue roasting for 15 minutes, or until the vegetables are fork-tender.
8. Divide the roasted vegetables between two plates and serve warm.

Nutrition Info:
- Per Serving: Calories: 333;Fat: 16.8g;Protein: 12.2g;-Carbs: 37.6g.

Paprika Cauliflower Steaks With Walnut Sauce

Servings:2
Cooking Time: 30 Minutes

Ingredients:
- Walnut Sauce:
- ½ cup raw walnut halves
- 2 tablespoons virgin olive oil, divided
- 1 clove garlic, chopped
- 1 small yellow onion, chopped
- ½ cup unsweetened almond milk
- 2 tablespoons fresh lemon juice
- Salt and pepper, to taste
- Paprika Cauliflower:
- 1 medium head cauliflower
- 1 teaspoon sweet paprika
- 1 teaspoon minced fresh thyme leaves

Directions:
1. Preheat the oven to 350°F.
2. Make the walnut sauce: Toast the walnuts in a large, ovenproof skillet over medium heat until fragrant and slightly darkened, about 5 minutes. Transfer the walnuts to a blender.
3. Heat 1 tablespoon of olive oil in the skillet. Add the garlic and onion and sauté for about 2 minutes, or until slightly softened. Transfer the garlic and onion into the blender, along with the almond milk, lemon juice, salt, and pepper. Blend the ingredients until smooth and creamy. Keep the sauce warm while you prepare the cauliflower.
4. Make the paprika cauliflower: Cut two 1-inch-thick "steaks" from the center of the cauliflower. Lightly moisten the steaks with water and season both sides with paprika, thyme, salt, and pepper.
5. Heat the remaining 1 tablespoon of olive oil in the skillet over medium-high heat. Add the cauliflower steaks and sear for about 3 minutes until evenly browned. Flip the cauliflower steaks and transfer the skillet to the oven.
6. Roast in the preheated oven for about 20 minutes until crisp-tender.
7. Serve the cauliflower steaks warm with the walnut sauce on the side.

Nutrition Info:
- Per Serving: Calories: 367;Fat: 27.9g;Protein: 7.0g;-Carbs: 22.7g.

Roasted Veggies And Brown Rice Bowl

Servings:4
Cooking Time: 20 Minutes

Ingredients:
- 2 cups cauliflower florets
- 2 cups broccoli florets
- 1 can chickpeas, drained and rinsed
- 1 cup carrot slices
- 2 to 3 tablespoons extra-virgin olive oil, divided
- Salt and freshly ground black pepper, to taste
- Nonstick cooking spray
- 2 cups cooked brown rice
- 2 to 3 tablespoons sesame seeds, for garnish
- Dressing:
- 3 to 4 tablespoons tahini
- 2 tablespoons honey
- 1 lemon, juiced
- 1 garlic clove, minced
- Salt and freshly ground black pepper, to taste

Directions:
1. Preheat the oven to 400°F. Spritz two baking sheets with nonstick cooking spray.
2. Spread the cauliflower and broccoli on the first baking sheet and the second with the chickpeas and carrot slices.
3. Drizzle each sheet with half of the olive oil and sprinkle with salt and pepper. Toss to coat well.
4. Roast the chickpeas and carrot slices in the preheated oven for 10 minutes, leaving the carrots tender but crisp, and the cauliflower and broccoli for 20 minutes until fork-tender. Stir them once halfway through the cooking time.
5. Meanwhile, make the dressing: Whisk together the tahini, honey, lemon juice, garlic, salt, and pepper in a small bowl.
6. Divide the cooked brown rice among four bowls. Top each bowl evenly with roasted vegetables and dressing. Sprinkle the sesame seeds on top for garnish before serving.

Nutrition Info:
- Per Serving: Calories: 453;Fat: 17.8g;Protein: 12.1g;-Carbs: 61.8g.

Stir-fried Kale With Mushrooms

Servings:4
Cooking Time:10 Minutes

Ingredients:
- 1 cup cremini mushrooms, sliced
- 4 tbsp olive oil
- 1 small red onion, chopped
- 2 cloves garlic, thinly sliced
- 1 ½ lb curly kale
- 2 tomatoes, chopped
- 1 tsp dried oregano
- 1 tsp dried basil
- ½ tsp dried rosemary
- ½ tsp dried thyme
- Salt and black pepper to taste

Directions:
1. Warm the olive oil in a saucepan over medium heat. Sauté the onion and garlic for about 3 minutes or until they are softened. Add in the mushrooms, kale, and tomatoes, stirring to promote even cooking. Turn the heat to a simmer, add in the spices and cook for 5-6 minutes until the kale wilt.

Nutrition Info:
- Per Serving: Calories: 221;Fat: 16g;Protein: 9g;Carbs: 19g.

Sautéed Spinach And Leeks

Servings:2
Cooking Time: 8 Minutes

Ingredients:
- 3 tablespoons olive oil
- 2 garlic cloves, crushed
- 2 leeks, chopped
- 2 red onions, chopped
- 9 ounces fresh spinach
- 1 teaspoon kosher salt
- ½ cup crumbled goat cheese

Directions:
1. Coat the bottom of the Instant Pot with the olive oil.
2. Add the garlic, leek, and onions and stir-fry for about 5 minutes, on Sauté mode.
3. Stir in the spinach. Sprinkle with the salt and sauté for an additional 3 minutes, stirring constantly.
4. Transfer to a plate and scatter with the goat cheese before serving.

Nutrition Info:
- Per Serving: Calories: 447;Fat: 31.2g;Protein: 14.6g;-Carbs: 28.7g.

Grilled Za´atar Zucchini Rounds

Servings:4
Cooking Time:20 Minutes

Ingredients:
- 2 tbsp olive oil
- 4 zucchinis, sliced
- 1 tbsp za'atar seasoning
- Salt to taste
- 2 tbsp parsley, chopped

Directions:
1. Preheat the grill on high. Cut the zucchini lengthways into ½-inch thin pieces. Brush the zucchini 'steaks' with olive oil and season with salt and za'atar seasoning. Grill for 6 minutes on both sides. Sprinkle with parsley and serve.

Nutrition Info:
- Per Serving: Calories: 91;Fat: 7.4g;Protein: 2.4g;Carbs: 6.6g.

Grilled Romaine Lettuce

Servings:4
Cooking Time: 3 To 5 Minutes

Ingredients:
- Romaine:
- 2 heads romaine lettuce, halved lengthwise
- 2 tablespoons extra-virgin olive oil
- Dressing:
- ½ cup unsweetened almond milk
- 1 tablespoon extra-virgin olive oil
- ¼ bunch fresh chives, thinly chopped
- 1 garlic clove, pressed
- 1 pinch red pepper flakes

Directions:
1. Heat a grill pan over medium heat.
2. Brush each lettuce half with the olive oil. Place the lettuce halves, flat-side down, on the grill. Grill for 3 to 5 minutes, or until the lettuce slightly wilts and develops light grill marks.
3. Meanwhile, whisk together all the ingredients for the dressing in a small bowl.
4. Drizzle 2 tablespoons of the dressing over each romaine half and serve.

Nutrition Info:
- Per Serving: Calories: 126;Fat: 11.0g;Protein: 2.0g;-Carbs: 7.0g.

Vegetable And Tofu Scramble

Servings:2
Cooking Time: 10 Minutes

Ingredients:
- 2 tablespoons extra-virgin olive oil
- ½ red onion, finely chopped
- 1 cup chopped kale
- 8 ounces mushrooms, sliced
- 8 ounces tofu, cut into pieces
- 2 garlic cloves, minced
- Pinch red pepper flakes
- ½ teaspoon sea salt
- ⅛ teaspoon freshly ground black pepper

Directions:
1. Heat the olive oil in a medium nonstick skillet over medium-high heat until shimmering.
2. Add the onion, kale, and mushrooms to the skillet and cook for about 5 minutes, stirring occasionally, or until the vegetables start to brown.
3. Add the tofu and stir-fry for 3 to 4 minutes until softened.
4. Stir in the garlic, red pepper flakes, salt, and black pepper and cook for 30 seconds.
5. Let the mixture cool for 5 minutes before serving.

Nutrition Info:
- Per Serving: Calories: 233;Fat: 15.9g;Protein: 13.4g;-Carbs: 11.9g.

Garlicky Zucchini Cubes With Mint

Servings:4
Cooking Time: 10 Minutes

Ingredients:
- 3 large green zucchinis, cut into ½-inch cubes
- 3 tablespoons extra-virgin olive oil
- 1 large onion, chopped
- 3 cloves garlic, minced
- 1 teaspoon salt
- 1 teaspoon dried mint

Directions:
1. Heat the olive oil in a large skillet over medium heat.
2. Add the onion and garlic and sauté for 3 minutes, stirring constantly, or until softened.
3. Stir in the zucchini cubes and salt and cook for 5 minutes, or until the zucchini is browned and tender.
4. Add the mint to the skillet and toss to combine, then continue cooking for 2 minutes.
5. Serve warm.

Nutrition Info:
- Per Serving: Calories: 146;Fat: 10.6g;Protein: 4.2g;-Carbs: 11.8g.

Creamy Polenta With Mushrooms

Servings:2
Cooking Time: 30 Minutes

Ingredients:
- ½ ounce dried porcini mushrooms (optional but recommended)
- 2 tablespoons olive oil
- 1 pound baby bella (cremini) mushrooms, quartered
- 1 large shallot, minced
- 1 garlic clove, minced
- 1 tablespoon flour
- 2 teaspoons tomato paste
- ½ cup red wine
- 1 cup mushroom stock (or reserved liquid from soaking the porcini mushrooms, if using)
- ½ teaspoon dried thyme
- 1 fresh rosemary sprig
- 1½ cups water
- ½ teaspoon salt
- ⅓ cup instant polenta
- 2 tablespoons grated Parmesan cheese

Directions:
1. If using the dried porcini mushrooms, soak them in 1 cup of hot water for about 15 minutes to soften them. When they're softened, scoop them out of the water, reserving the soaking liquid. Mince the porcini mushrooms.
2. Heat the olive oil in a large sauté pan over medium-high heat. Add the mushrooms, shallot, and garlic, and sauté for 10 minutes, or until the vegetables are wilted and starting to caramelize.
3. Add the flour and tomato paste, and cook for another 30 seconds. Add the red wine, mushroom stock or porcini soaking liquid, thyme, and rosemary. Bring the mixture to a boil, stirring constantly until it thickens. Reduce the heat and let it simmer for 10 minutes.
4. Meanwhile, bring the water to a boil in a saucepan and add salt.
5. Add the instant polenta and stir quickly while it thickens. Stir in the Parmesan cheese. Taste and add additional salt, if needed. Serve warm.

Nutrition Info:
- Per Serving: Calories: 450;Fat: 16.0g;Protein: 14.1g;-Carbs: 57.8g.

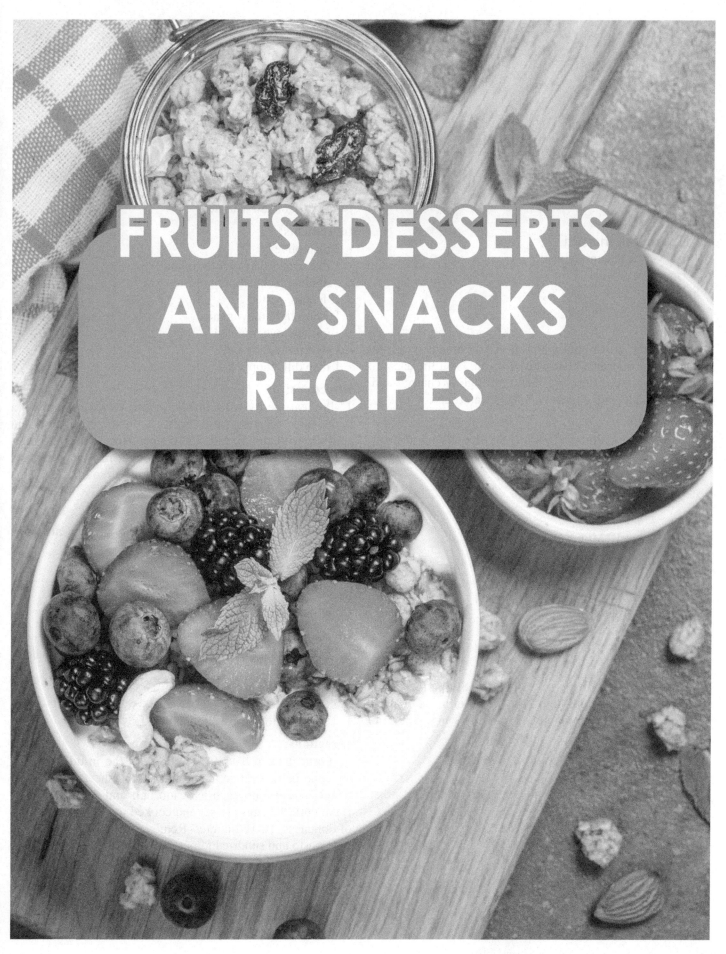

FRUITS, DESSERTS AND SNACKS RECIPES

Charred Asparagus

Servings:4
Cooking Time:25 Minutes

Ingredients:
- 2 tbsp olive oil
- 1 lb asparagus, trimmed
- 4 tbsp Grana Padano, grated
- ½ tsp garlic powder
- Salt to taste
- 2 tbsp parsley, chopped

Directions:
1. Preheat the grill to high. Season the asparagus with salt and garlic powder and coat with olive oil. Grill the asparagus for 10 minutes, turning often until lightly charred and tender. Sprinkle with cheese and parsley and serve.

Nutrition Info:
- Per Serving: Calories: 105;Fat: 8g;Protein: 4.3g;Carbs: 4.7g.

Simple Apple Compote

Servings:4
Cooking Time: 10 Minutes

Ingredients:
- 6 apples, peeled, cored, and chopped
- ¼ cup raw honey
- 1 teaspoon ground cinnamon
- ¼ cup apple juice
- Sea salt, to taste

Directions:
1. Put all the ingredients in a stockpot. Stir to mix well, then cook over medium-high heat for 10 minutes or until the apples are glazed by honey and lightly saucy. Stir constantly.
2. Serve immediately.

Nutrition Info:
- Per Serving: Calories: 246;Fat: 0.9g;Protein: 1.2g;Carbs: 66.3g.

Roasted Carrot Ribbons With Mayo Sauce

Servings:4
Cooking Time:50 Minutes

Ingredients:
- 2 tbsp olive oil
- 1 lb carrots, shaved into ribbons
- Salt and black pepper to taste
- ½ lemon, zested
- 1/3 cup light mayonnaise
- 1 garlic clove, minced
- 1 tsp cumin, ground
- 1 tbsp dill, chopped

Directions:
1. Preheat the oven to 380 F. Spread carrot ribbons on a paper-lined roasting tray. Drizzle with some olive oil and sprinkle with cumin, salt, and pepper. Roast for 20-25 minutes until crisp and golden. In a bowl, mix mayonnaise, lemon zest, garlic, dill, and remaining olive oil. Serve the roasted carrots with mayo sauce.

Nutrition Info:
- Per Serving: Calories: 200;Fat: 6g;Protein: 6g;Carbs: 8g.

Pesto & Egg Avocado Boats

Servings:2
Cooking Time:15 Minutes

Ingredients:
- 1 halved avocado, pitted
- 2 large eggs
- Salt and black pepper to taste
- 2 tbsp jarred pesto
- 2 sundried tomatoes, chopped

Directions:
1. Preheat oven to 420 F. Scoop out the middle of each avocado half. Arrange them on a baking sheet, cut-side up. Crack an egg into each avocado half and season to taste. Bake until the eggs are set and cooked to your desired level of doneness, 10-12 minutes. Remove from the oven and top with pesto and sundried tomatoes. Serve and enjoy!

Nutrition Info:
- Per Serving: Calories: 302;Fat: 26g;Protein: 8g;Carbs: 10g.

Frozen Mango Raspberry Delight

Servings:2
Cooking Time: 0 Minutes

Ingredients:
- 3 cups frozen raspberries
- 1 mango, peeled and pitted
- 1 peach, peeled and pitted
- 1 teaspoon honey

Directions:
1. Place all the ingredients into a blender and purée, adding some water as needed.
2. Put in the freezer for 10 minutes to firm up if desired. Serve chilled or at room temperature.

Nutrition Info:
- Per Serving: Calories: 276;Fat: 2.1g;Protein: 4.5g;Carbs: 60.3g.

Turkish Dolma (stuffed Grape Leaves)

Servings:4
Cooking Time:50 Minutes

Ingredients:
- 2 tbsp olive oil
- 1 onion, chopped
- 2 garlic cloves, minced
- 1 cup short-grain rice
- ¼ cup gold raisins
- ¼ cup pine nuts, toasted
- 1 lemon, juiced
- ¼ tsp ground cinnamon
- Salt and black pepper to taste
- 2 tbsp parsley, chopped
- 20 preserved grape leaves

Directions:
1. Warm the olive oil in a skillet over medium heat. Add the onion and garlic and sauté for 5 minutes. Add the rice, golden raisins, pine nuts, cinnamon, and lemon juice. Season with salt and pepper. Stuff each leaf with about 1 tablespoon of the filling. Roll tightly and place each in a pot, seam side down. Add 2 cups of water and simmer for about 15-18 minutes. Serve warm.

Nutrition Info:
- Per Serving: Calories: 237;Fat: 12g;Protein: 7g;Carbs: 26g.

Pesto Arugula Dip

Servings:4
Cooking Time:5 Minutes

Ingredients:
- 1 cup arugula, chopped
- 3 tbsp basil pesto
- 1 cup cream cheese, soft
- Salt and black pepper to taste
- 1 cup heavy cream
- 1 tbsp chives, chopped

Directions:
1. Combine arugula, basil pesto, salt, pepper, and heavy cream in a blender and pulse until smooth. Transfer to a bowl and mix in cream cheese. Serve topped with chives.

Nutrition Info:
- Per Serving: Calories: 240;Fat: 15g;Protein: 6g;Carbs: 7g.

Chickpea & Spinach Salad With Almonds

Servings:4
Cooking Time:5 Minutes

Ingredients:
- 2 tbsp olive oil
- 3 spring onions, chopped
- 1 cup baby spinach
- 15 oz canned chickpeas
- Salt and black pepper to taste
- 2 tbsp lemon juice
- 1 tbsp cilantro, chopped
- 2 tbsp almonds flakes, toasted

Directions:
1. Toss chickpeas, spring onions, spinach, salt, pepper, olive oil, lemon juice, and cilantro in a salad bowl. Top with almond flakes. Serve and enjoy!

Nutrition Info:
- Per Serving: Calories: 230;Fat: 6g;Protein: 16g;Carbs: 10g.

Turkey Pesto Pizza

Servings:4
Cooking Time:35 Minutes

Ingredients:
- Pizza Crust
- 3 tbsp olive oil
- 3 cups flour
- ¼ tsp salt
- 3 large eggs
- Topping
- ½ lb turkey ham, chopped
- 2 tbsp cashew nuts
- 1 green bell pepper, sliced
- 1 ½ cups basil pesto
- 1 cup mozzarella, grated
- 2 tbsp Parmesan cheese, grated
- 4 fresh basil leaves, chopped
- ¼ tsp red pepper flakes

Directions:
1. In a bowl, mix flour, olive oil, salt, and egg until a dough forms. Mold the dough into a ball and place it in between two full parchment papers on a flat surface. Roll it out into a circle of a ¼ -inch thickness. After, slide the pizza dough into the pizza pan and remove the parchment paper. Place the pizza pan in the oven and bake the dough for 20 minutes at 350 F. Once the pizza bread is ready, remove it from the oven, fold and seal the extra inch of dough at its edges to make a crust around it. Apply 2/3 of the pesto on it and sprinkle half of the mozzarella cheese too.

2. Toss the chopped turkey ham in the remaining pesto and spread it on top of the pizza. Sprinkle with the remaining mozzarella, bell peppers, and cashew nuts and put the pizza back in the oven to bake for 9 minutes. When it is ready, remove from the oven to cool slightly, garnish with the basil leaves and sprinkle with parmesan cheese and red pepper flakes. Slice and serve.

Nutrition Info:
- Per Serving: Calories: 684;Fat: 54g;Protein: 32g;Carbs: 22g.

Lovely Coconut-covered Strawberries

Servings:4
Cooking Time:15 Min + Cooling Time

Ingredients:
- 1 cup chocolate chips
- ¼ cup coconut flakes
- 1 lb strawberries
- ½ tsp vanilla extract
- ½ tsp ground nutmeg
- ¼ tsp salt

Directions:

1. Melt chocolate chips for 30 seconds. Remove and stir in vanilla, nutmeg, and salt. Let cool for 2-3 minutes. Dip strawberries into the chocolate and then into the coconut flakes. Place on a wax paper-lined cookie sheet and let sit for 30 minutes until the chocolate dries. Serve.

Nutrition Info:
- Per Serving: Calories: 275;Fat: 20g;Protein: 6g;Carbs: 21g.

Artichoke & Sun-dried Tomato Pizza

Servings:4
Cooking Time:80 Minutes

Ingredients:
- 2 tbsp olive oil
- 1 cup canned passata
- 2 cups flour
- 1 pinch of sugar
- 1 tsp active dry yeast
- ¾ tsp salt
- 1 ½ cups artichoke hearts
- ¼ cup grated Asiago cheese
- ½ onion, minced
- 3 garlic cloves, minced
- 1 tbsp dried oregano
- 6 sundried tomatoes, chopped
- ½ tsp red pepper flakes
- 5-6 basil leaves, torn

Directions:
1. Sift the flour and salt in a bowl and stir in yeast. Mix 1 cup of lukewarm water, olive oil, and sugar in another bowl. Add the wet mixture to the dry mixture and whisk until you obtain a soft dough. Place the dough on a lightly floured work surface and knead it thoroughly for 4-5 minutes until elastic. Transfer the dough to a greased bowl. Cover with cling film and leave to rise for 50-60 minutes in a warm place until doubled in size. Roll out the dough to a thickness of around 12 inches.

2. Preheat oven to 400 F. Warm oil in a saucepan over medium heat and sauté onion and garlic for 3-4 minutes. Mix in tomatoes and oregano and bring to a boil. Decrease the heat and simmer for another 5 minutes. Transfer the pizza crust to a baking sheet. Spread the sauce all over and top with artichoke hearts and sun-dried tomatoes. Scatter the cheese and bake for 15 minutes until golden. Top with red pepper flakes and basil leaves and serve sliced.

Nutrition Info:
- Per Serving: Calories: 254;Fat: 9.5g;Protein: 8g;Carbs: 34.3g.

Caramel Peach & Walnut Cake

Servings:6
Cooking Time:50 Min + Cooling Time

Ingredients:
- ¼ cup coconut oil
- ¼ cup olive oil
- 2 peeled peaches, chopped
- ½ cup raisins, soaked
- 1 cup plain flour
- 3 eggs
- 1 tbsp dark rum
- ¼ tsp ground cinnamon
- 1 tsp vanilla extract
- 1 ½ tsp baking powder
- 4 tbsp Greek yogurt
- 2 tbsp honey
- 1 cup brown sugar
- 4 tbsp walnuts, chopped
- ¼ caramel sauce
- ¼ tsp salt

Directions:
1. Preheat the oven to 350 F. In a bowl, mix the flour, cinnamon, vanilla, baking powder, and salt. In another bowl, whisk the eggs with Greek yogurt using an electric mixer. Gently add in coconut and olive oil. Combine well. Put in rum, honey and sugar; stir to combine. Mix the wet ingredients with the dry mixture. Stir in peaches, raisins, and walnuts.
2. Pour the mixture into a greased baking pan and bake for 30-40 minutes until a knife inserted into the middle of the cake comes out clean. Remove from the oven and let sit for 10 minutes, then invert onto a wire rack to cool completely. Warm the caramel sauce through in a pan and pour it over the cooled cake to serve.

Nutrition Info:
- Per Serving: Calories: 568;Fat: 26g;Protein: 215g;Carbs: 66g.

Fruit Skewers With Vanilla Labneh

Servings:4
Cooking Time:15 Min + Straining Time

Ingredients:
- 2 cups plain yogurt
- 2 tbsp honey
- 1 tsp vanilla extract
- A pinch of salt
- 2 mangoes, cut into chunks

Directions:
1. Place a fine sieve lined with cheesecloth over a bowl and spoon the yogurt into the sieve. Allow the liquid to drain off for 12-24 hours hours. Transfer the strained yogurt to a bowl and mix in the honey, vanilla, and salt. Set it aside.
2. Heat your grill to medium-high. Thread the fruit onto skewers and grill for 2 minutes on each side until the fruit is softened and has grill marks on each side. Serve with labneh.

Nutrition Info:
- Per Serving: Calories: 292;Fat: 6g;Protein: 5g;Carbs: 60g.

Avocado & Salmon Stuffed Cucumbers

Servings:4
Cooking Time:10 Minutes

Ingredients:
- 1 tbsp extra-virgin olive oil
- 2 large cucumbers, peeled
- 1 can red salmon
- 1 ripe avocado, mashed
- 2 tbsp chopped fresh dill
- Salt and black pepper to taste

Directions:
1. Cut the cucumber into 1-inch-thick segments, and using a spoon, scrape seeds out of the center of each piece and stand up on a plate. In a bowl, mix the salmon, avocado, olive oil, lime zest and juice, dill, salt, and pepper, and blend until creamy. Spoon the salmon mixture into the center of each cucumber segment and serve chilled.

Nutrition Info:
- Per Serving: Calories: 159;Fat: 11g;Protein: 9g;Carbs: 8g.

Italian Popcorn

Servings:6
Cooking Time:20 Minutes

Ingredients:
- 2 tbsp butter, melted
- 1 tbsp truffle oil
- 8 cups air-popped popcorn
- 2 tbsp packed brown sugar
- 2 tbsp Italian seasoning
- ¼ tsp sea salt

Directions:
1. Preheat oven to 350 F. Combine butter, Italian seasoning, sugar, and salt in a bowl. Pour over the popcorn and toss well to coat. Remove to a baking dish and bake for 15 minutes, stirring frequently. Drizzle with truffle oil and serve.

Nutrition Info:
- Per Serving: Calories: 80;Fat: 5g;Protein: 1.1g;Carbs: 8.4g.

Olive Mezze Platter

Servings:2
Cooking Time:10 Min + Marinating Time

Ingredients:
- 2 cups mixed green olives with pits
- ¼ cup extra-virgin olive oil
- ¼ cup red wine vinegar
- 1 tsp dried oregano
- 1 orange, zested and juiced
- ½ tsp crushed chilies
- ½ tsp ground cumin

Directions:
1. Combine the olives, vinegar, olive oil, garlic, oregano, crushed chilies, and cumin in a large glass and mix well. Cover and set aside to marinate for 30 minutes. Keep for up to 14 days in the refrigerator.

Nutrition Info:
- Per Serving: Calories: 133;Fat: 14g;Protein: 1g;Carbs: 3g.

Dark Chocolate Barks

Servings:6
Cooking Time:20 Min + Freezing Time

Ingredients:
- ½ cup quinoa
- ½ tsp sea salt
- 1 cup dark chocolate chips
- ½ tsp mint extract
- ½ cup pomegranate seeds

Directions:
1. Toast the quinoa in a greased saucepan for 2-3 minutes, stirring frequently. Remove the pan from the stove and mix in the salt. Set aside 2 tablespoons of the toasted quinoa.
2. Microwave the chocolate for 1 minute. Stir until the chocolate is completely melted. Mix the toasted quinoa and mint extract into the melted chocolate. Line a large, rimmed baking sheet with parchment paper. Spread the chocolate mixture onto the sheet. Sprinkle the remaining 2 tablespoons of quinoa and pomegranate seeds, pressing with a spatula. Freeze the mixture for 10-15 minutes or until set. Remove and break into about 2-inch jagged pieces. Store in the refrigerator until ready to serve.

Nutrition Info:
- Per Serving: Calories: 268;Fat: 12g;Protein: 4g;Carbs: 37g.

Spiced Nut Mix

Servings:6
Cooking Time:20 Minutes

Ingredients:
- 1 tbsp olive oil
- 2 cups raw mixed nuts
- 1 tsp ground cumin
- ½ tsp garlic powder
- ½ tsp kosher salt
- ⅛ tsp chili powder
- ⅛ tsp ground coriander

Directions:
1. Place the nuts in a skillet over medium heat and toast for 3 minutes, shaking the pan continuously. Remove to a bowl, season with salt, and reserve. Warm olive oil in the same skillet. Add in cumin, garlic powder, chili powder, and ground coriander and cook for about 20-30 seconds. Mix in nuts and cook for another 4 minutes. Serve chilled.

Nutrition Info:
- Per Serving: Calories: 315;Fat: 29.2g;Protein: 8g;Carbs: 11g.

Roasted Garlic & Spicy Lentil Dip

Servings:6
Cooking Time:40 Minutes

Ingredients:
- 1 roasted red bell pepper, chopped
- 4 tbsp olive oil
- 1 cup split red lentils
- ½ red onion
- 1 garlic bulb, top removed
- ½ tsp cumin seeds
- 1 tsp coriander seeds
- ¼ cup walnuts
- 2 tbsp tomato paste
- ½ tsp Cayenne powder
- Salt and black pepper to taste

Directions:
1. Preheat oven to 370 F. Drizzle the garlic with some olive oil and wrap it in a piece of aluminum foil. Roast for 35-40 minutes. Remove and allow to cool for a few minutes. Cover the lentils with salted water in a pot over medium heat and bring to a boil. Simmer for 15 minutes. Drain and set aside.
2. Squeeze out the garlic cloves and place them in a food processor. Add in the cooled lentils, cumin seeds, coriander seeds, roasted red bell pepper, onion, walnuts, tomato paste, Cayenne powder, remaining olive oil, salt, and black pepper. Pulse until smooth. Serve with crostiniif desire.

Nutrition Info:
- Per Serving: Calories: 234;Fat: 13g;Protein: 9g;Carbs: 21.7g.

Coconut Blueberries With Brown Rice

Servings:4
Cooking Time: 10 Minutes

Ingredients:
- 1 cup fresh blueberries
- 2 cups unsweetened coconut milk
- 1 teaspoon ground ginger
- ¼ cup maple syrup
- Sea salt, to taste
- 2 cups cooked brown rice

Directions:
1. Put all the ingredients, except for the brown rice, in a pot. Stir to combine well.
2. Cook over medium-high heat for 7 minutes or until the blueberries are tender.
3. Pour in the brown rice and cook for 3 more minute or until the rice is soft. Stir constantly.
4. Serve immediately.

Nutrition Info:
- Per Serving: Calories: 470;Fat: 24.8g;Protein: 6.2g;-Carbs: 60.1g.

Simple Spiced Sweet Pecans

Servings:4
Cooking Time: 17 Minutes

Ingredients:
- 1 cup pecan halves
- 3 tablespoons almond butter
- 1 teaspoon ground cinnamon
- ½ teaspoon ground nutmeg
- ¼ cup raw honey
- ¼ teaspoon sea salt

Directions:
1. Preheat the oven to 350ºF. Line a baking sheet with parchment paper.
2. Combine all the ingredients in a bowl. Stir to mix well, then spread the mixture in the single layer on the baking sheet with a spatula.
3. Bake in the preheated oven for 16 minutes or until the pecan halves are well browned.
4. Serve immediately.

Nutrition Info:
- Per Serving: Calories: 324;Fat: 29.8g;Protein: 3.2g;-Carbs: 13.9g.

Lemony Blackberry Granita

Servings:4
Cooking Time: 0 Minutes

Ingredients:
- 1 pound fresh blackberries
- 1 teaspoon chopped fresh thyme
- ¼ cup freshly squeezed lemon juice
- ½ cup raw honey
- ½ cup water

Directions:
1. Put all the ingredients in a food processor, then pulse to purée.
2. Pour the mixture through a sieve into a baking dish. Discard the seeds remain in the sieve.
3. Put the baking dish in the freezer for 2 hours. Remove the dish from the refrigerator and stir to break any frozen parts.
4. Return the dish back to the freezer for an hour, then stir to break any frozen parts again.
5. Return the dish to the freezer for 4 hours until the granita is completely frozen.
6. Remove it from the freezer and mash to serve.

Nutrition Info:
- Per Serving: Calories: 183;Fat: 1.1g;Protein: 2.2g;Carbs: 45.9g.

Mushroom & Black Olive Pizza

Servings:4
Cooking Time:45 Minutes

Ingredients:
- For the crust
- 2 tbsp olive oil
- 2 cups flour
- 1 cup lukewarm water
- 1 pinch of sugar
- 1 tsp active dry yeast
- ¾ tsp salt
- For the topping
- 2 medium cremini mushrooms, sliced
- 1 tsp olive oil
- 1 garlic clove, minced
- ½ cup tomato sauce
- 1 tsp sugar
- 1 bay leaf
- 1 tsp dried oregano
- 1tsp dried basil
- Salt and black pepper to taste
- ½ cup grated mozzarella
- ½ cup grated Parmesan cheese
- 6 black olives, sliced

Directions:
1. Sift the flour and salt in a bowl and stir in yeast. Mix lukewarm water, olive oil, and sugar in another bowl. Add the wet mixture to the dry mixture and whisk until you obtain a soft dough. Place the dough on a lightly floured work surface and knead it thoroughly for 4-5 minutes until elastic. Transfer the dough to a greased bowl. Cover with cling film and leave to rise for 50-60 minutes in a warm place until doubled in size. Roll out the dough to a thickness of around 12 inches.
2. Preheat the oven to 400 F. Line a pizza pan with parchment paper. Heat the olive oil in a medium skillet and sauté the mushrooms until softened, 5 minutes. Stir in the garlic and cook until fragrant, 30 seconds.
3. Mix in the tomato sauce, sugar, bay leaf, oregano, basil, salt, and black pepper. Cook for 2 minutes and turn the heat off. Spread the sauce on the crust, top with the mozzarella and Parmesan cheeses, and then, the olives. Bake in the oven until the cheeses melts, 15 minutes. Serve warm.

Nutrition Info:
- Per Serving: Calories: 203;Fat: 9g;Protein: 24g;Carbs: 2.6g.

Pepperoni Fat Head Pizza

Servings:4
Cooking Time:35 Minutes

Ingredients:
- 2 tbsp olive oil
- 2 cups flour
- 1 cup lukewarm water
- 1 pinch of sugar
- 1 tsp active dry yeast
- ¾ tsp salt
- 1 tsp dried oregano
- 2 cups mozzarella cheese
- 1 cup sliced pepperoni

Directions:
1. Sift the flour and salt in a bowl and stir in yeast. Mix lukewarm water, olive oil, and sugar in another bowl. Add the wet mixture to the dry mixture and whisk until you obtain a soft dough. Place the dough on a lightly floured work surface and knead it thoroughly for 4-5 minutes until elastic. Transfer the dough to a greased bowl. Cover with cling film and leave to rise for 50-60 minutes in a warm place until doubled in size. Roll out the dough to a thickness of around 12 inches.
2. Preheat oven to 400 F. Line a round pizza pan with parchment paper. Spread the dough on the pizza pan and top with the mozzarella cheese, oregano, and pepperoni slices. Bake in the oven for 15 minutes or until the cheese melts. Remove the pizza from the oven and let cool slightly. Slice and serve.

Nutrition Info:
- Per Serving: Calories: 229;Fat: 7g;Protein: 36g;Carbs: 0.4g.

Mint-watermelon Gelato

Servings:4
Cooking Time:10 Min + Freezing Time

Ingredients:
- ¼ cup honey
- 4 cups watermelon cubes
- ¼ cup lemon juice
- 12 mint leaves to serve

Directions:
1. In a food processor, blend the watermelon, honey, and lemon juice to form a purée with chunks. Transfer to a freezer-proof container and place in the freezer for 1 hour.
2. Remove the container from and scrape with a fork. Return the to the freezer and repeat the process every half hour until the sorbet is completely frozen, for around 4 hours. Share into bowls, garnish with mint leaves, and serve.

Nutrition Info:
- Per Serving: Calories: 149;Fat: 0.4g;Protein: 1.8g;Carbs: 38g.

Home-style Trail Mix

Servings:4
Cooking Time:30 Minutes

Ingredients:
- 1 cup dried apricots, cut into thin strips
- 2 tbsp olive oil
- 1 cup pepitas
- 1 cup walnut halves
- 1 cup dried dates, chopped
- 1 cup golden raisins
- 1 cup raw almonds
- 1 tsp salt

Directions:
1. Preheat the oven to 310 F. Combine almonds, pepitas, dates, walnuts, apricots, and raisins in a bowl. Mix in olive oil and salt and toss to coat. Spread the mixture on a lined with parchment paper sheet, and bake for 30 minutes or until the fruits are slightly browned. Let to cool before serving.

Nutrition Info:
- Per Serving: Calories: 267;Fat: 14g;Protein: 7g;Carbs: 35g.

Eggplant & Bell Pepper Spread

Servings:4
Cooking Time:55 Minutes

Ingredients:
- ¼ cup olive oil
- 1 cup light mayonnaise
- 2 eggplants, sliced
- Salt and black pepper to taste
- 4 garlic cloves, minced
- 1 tbsp chives, chopped

Directions:
1. Preheat the oven to 360 F. Arrange bell peppers and eggplants on a baking pan. Sprinkle with salt, pepper, and garlic and drizzle with some olive oil. Bake for 45 minutes. Transfer to a food processor and pulse until smooth a few times while gradually adding the remaining olive oil. Remove to a bowl and mix in mayonnaise. Top with chives and serve.

Nutrition Info:
- Per Serving: Calories: 220;Fat: 14g;Protein: 4g;Carbs: 25g.

Chocolate And Avocado Mousse

Servings:4
Cooking Time: 5 Minutes

Ingredients:
- 8 ounces dark chocolate, chopped
- ¼ cup unsweetened coconut milk
- 2 tablespoons coconut oil
- 2 ripe avocados, deseeded
- ¼ cup raw honey
- Sea salt, to taste

Directions:
1. Put the chocolate in a saucepan. Pour in the coconut milk and add the coconut oil.
2. Cook for 3 minutes or until the chocolate and coconut oil melt. Stir constantly.
3. Put the avocado in a food processor, then drizzle with honey and melted chocolate. Pulse to combine until smooth.
4. Pour the mixture in a serving bowl, then sprinkle with salt. Refrigerate to chill for 30 minutes and serve.

Nutrition Info:
- Per Serving: Calories: 654;Fat: 46.8g;Protein: 7.2g;-Carbs: 55.9g.

Raspberry Yogurt Basted Cantaloupe

Servings:6
Cooking Time: 0 Minutes

Ingredients:
- 2 cups fresh raspberries, mashed
- 1 cup plain coconut yogurt
- ½ teaspoon vanilla extract
- 1 cantaloupe, peeled and sliced
- ½ cup toasted coconut flakes

Directions:
1. Combine the mashed raspberries with yogurt and vanilla extract in a small bowl. Stir to mix well.
2. Place the cantaloupe slices on a platter, then top with raspberry mixture and spread with toasted coconut.
3. Serve immediately.

Nutrition Info:
- Per Serving: Calories: 75;Fat: 4.1g;Protein: 1.2g;Carbs: 10.9g.

Two-cheese Stuffed Bell Peppers

Servings:6
Cooking Time:20 Min + Chilling Time

Ingredients:
- 1 ½ lb bell peppers, cored and seeded
- 1 tbsp extra-virgin olive oil
- 4 oz ricotta cheese
- 4 oz mascarpone cheese
- 1 tbsp scallions, chopped
- 1 tbsp lemon zest

Directions:
1. Preheat oven to 400 F. Coat the peppers with olive oil, put them on a baking sheet, and roast for 8 minutes. Remove and let cool. In a bowl, add the ricotta cheese, mascarpone cheese, scallions, and lemon zest. Stir to combine, then spoon mixture into a piping bag. Stuff each pepper to the top with the cheese mixture. Chill the peppers and serve.

Nutrition Info:
- Per Serving: Calories: 141;Fat: 11g;Protein: 4g;Carbs: 6g.

Mint Raspberries Panna Cotta

Servings:4
Cooking Time:15 Min + Chilling Time

Ingredients:
- 2 tbsp warm water
- 2 tsp gelatin powder
- 2 cups heavy cream
- 1 cup raspberries
- 2 tbsp sugar
- 1 tsp vanilla extract
- 4 fresh mint leaves

Directions:
1. Pour 2 tbsp of warm water into a small bowl. Stir in the gelatin to dissolve. Allow the mixture to sit for 10 minutes. In a large bowl, combine the heavy cream, raspberries, sugar, and vanilla. Blend with an immersion blender until the mixture is smooth and the raspberries are well puréed. Transfer the mixture to a saucepan and heat over medium heat until just below a simmer. Remove from the heat and let cool for 5 minutes. Add in the gelatin mixture, whisking constantly until smooth. Divide the custard between ramekins and refrigerate until set, 4-6 hours. Serve chilled garnished with mint leaves.

Nutrition Info:
- Per Serving: Calories: 431;Fat: 44g;Protein: 4g;Carbs: 7g.

Spiced Hot Chocolate

Servings:4
Cooking Time:15 Minutes

Ingredients:
- ¼ tsp cayenne pepper powder
- 4 squares chocolate
- 4 cups milk
- 2 tsp sugar
- ½ tsp ground cinnamon
- ½ tsp salt

Directions:
1. Place milk and sugar in a pot over low heat and warm until it begins to simmer.
2. Combine chocolate, cinnamon, salt, and cayenne pepper powder in a bowl. Slowly pour in enough hot milk to cover. Return the pot to the heat and lower the temperature. Stir until the chocolate has melted, then add the remaining milk and combine. Spoon into 4 cups and serve hot.

Nutrition Info:
- Per Serving: Calories: 342;Fat: 23g;Protein: 12g;Carbs: 22g.

Berry Sorbet

Servings:4
Cooking Time:10 Min + Freezing Time

Ingredients:
- 1 tsp lemon juice
- ¼ cup honey
- 1 cup fresh strawberries
- 1 cup fresh raspberries
- 1 cup fresh blueberries

Directions:
1. Bring 1 cup of water to a boil in a pot over high heat. Stir in honey until dissolved. Remove from the heat and mix in berries and lemon juice; let cool.
2. Once cooled, add the mixture to a food processor and pulse until smooth. Transfer to a shallow glass and freeze for 1 hour. Stir with a fork and freeze for 30 more minutes. Repeat a couple of times. Serve in dessert dishes.

Nutrition Info:
- Per Serving: Calories: 115;Fat: 1g;Protein: 1g;Carbs: 29g.

Two Cheese Pizza

Servings:4
Cooking Time:35 Minutes

Ingredients:
- For the crust:
- 1 tbsp olive oil
- ½ cup almond flour
- ¼ tsp salt
- 2 tbsp ground psyllium husk
- For the topping
- ½ cup pizza sauce
- 4 oz mozzarella, sliced
- 1 cup grated mozzarella
- 3 tbsp grated Parmesan cheese
- 2 tsp Italian seasoning

Directions:
1. Preheat the oven to 400 F. Line a baking sheet with parchment paper. In a medium bowl, mix the almond flour, salt, psyllium powder, olive oil, and 1 cup of lukewarm water until dough forms. Spread the mixture on the pizza pan and bake in the oven until crusty, 10 minutes. When ready, remove the crust and spread the pizza sauce on top. Add the sliced mozzarella, grated mozzarella, Parmesan cheese, and Italian seasoning. Bake in the oven for 18 minutes or until the cheeses melt. Serve warm.

Nutrition Info:
- Per Serving: Calories: 193;Fat: 10g;Protein: 19g;Carbs: 3g.

Easy No-bake Walnut & Date Oat Bars

Servings:6
Cooking Time:30 Minutes

Ingredients:
- ¼ cup butter, melted
- ¼ cup honey
- 12 dates, pitted and chopped
- 1 tsp vanilla extract
- ½ cup rolled oats
- ¾ cup sultanas, soaked
- 1 cup walnuts, chopped
- ¼ cup pumpkin seeds

Directions:
1. Place dates, vanilla, honey, oats, sultanas, butter, walnuts, and pumpkin seeds in a bowl and mix to combine. Transfer to a lined with parchment paper baking sheet and freeze for 30 minutes. Slice into bars and serve.

Nutrition Info:
- Per Serving: Calories: 280;Fat: 14g;Protein: 4g;Carbs: 15g.

Glazed Pears With Hazelnuts

Servings:4
Cooking Time: 20 Minutes

Ingredients:
- 4 pears, peeled, cored, and quartered lengthwise
- 1 cup apple juice
- 1 tablespoon grated fresh ginger
- ½ cup pure maple syrup
- ¼ cup chopped hazelnuts

Directions:
1. Put the pears in a pot, then pour in the apple juice. Bring to a boil over medium-high heat, then reduce the heat to medium-low. Stir constantly.
2. Cover and simmer for an additional 15 minutes or until the pears are tender.
3. Meanwhile, combine the ginger and maple syrup in a saucepan. Bring to a boil over medium-high heat. Stir frequently. Turn off the heat and transfer the syrup to a small bowl and let sit until ready to use.
4. Transfer the pears in a large serving bowl with a slotted spoon, then top the pears with syrup.
5. Spread the hazelnuts over the pears and serve immediately.

Nutrition Info:
- Per Serving: Calories: 287;Fat: 3.1g;Protein: 2.2g;Carbs: 66.9g.

RECIPES

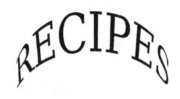

DATE

RECIPES	Salads	Meats	Soups
SERVES	Grains	Seafood	Snack
PREP TIME	Breads	Vegetables	Breakfast
COOK TIME	Appetizers	Desserts	Lunch
FROM THE KITCHEN OF	Main Dishes	Beverages	Dinners

INGREDIENTS

DIRECTIONS

NOTES

SERVING	☆☆☆☆☆
DIFFICULTY	☆☆☆☆☆
OVERALL	☆☆☆☆☆

Date: _____

MY SHOPPING LIST

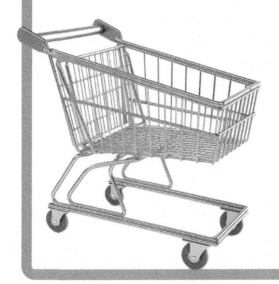

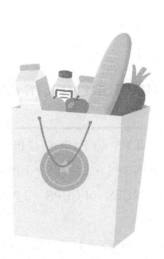

Appendix A : Measurement Conversions

BASIC KITCHEN CONVERSIONS & EQUIVALENTS

DRY MEASUREMENTS CONVERSION CHART

3 TEASPOONS = 1 TABLESPOON = 1/16 CUP

6 TEASPOONS = 2 TABLESPOONS = 1/8 CUP

12 TEASPOONS = 4 TABLESPOONS = 1/4 CUP

24 TEASPOONS = 8 TABLESPOONS = 1/2 CUP

36 TEASPOONS = 12 TABLESPOONS = 3/4 CUP

48 TEASPOONS = 16 TABLESPOONS = 1 CUP

METRIC TO US COOKING CONVERSIONS

OVEN TEMPERATURES

120 °C = 250 °F

160 °C = 320 °F

180° C = 350 °F

205 °C = 400 °F

220 °C = 425 °F

LIQUID MEASUREMENTS CONVERSION CHART

8 FLUID OUNCES = 1 CUP = 1/2 PINT = 1/4 QUART

16 FLUID OUNCES = 2 CUPS = 1 PINT = 1/2 QUART

32 FLUID OUNCES = 4 CUPS = 2 PINTS = 1 QUART
= 1/4 GALLON

128 FLUID OUNCES = 16 CUPS = 8 PINTS = 4 QUARTS
= 1 GALLON

BAKING IN GRAMS

1 CUP FLOUR = 140 GRAMS

1 CUP SUGAR = 150 GRAMS

1 CUP POWDERED SUGAR = 160 GRAMS

1 CUP HEAVY CREAM = 235 GRAMS

VOLUME

1 MILLILITER = 1/5 TEASPOON

5 ML = 1 TEASPOON

15 ML = 1 TABLESPOON

240 ML = 1 CUP OR 8 FLUID OUNCES

1 LITER = 34 FL. OUNCES

WEIGHT

1 GRAM = .035 OUNCES

100 GRAMS = 3.5 OUNCES

500 GRAMS = 1.1 POUNDS

1 KILOGRAM = 35 OUNCES

US TO METRIC COOKING CONVERSIONS

1/5 TSP = 1 ML

1 TSP = 5 ML

1 TBSP = 15 ML

1 FL OUNCE = 30 ML

1 CUP = 237 ML

1 PINT (2 CUPS) = 473 ML

1 QUART (4 CUPS) = .95 LITER

1 GALLON (16 CUPS) = 3.8 LITERS

1 OZ = 28 GRAMS

1 POUND = 454 GRAMS

BUTTER

1 CUP BUTTER = 2 STICKS = 8 OUNCES = 230 GRAMS = 8 TABLESPOONS

WHAT DOES 1 CUP EQUAL

1 CUP = 8 FLUID OUNCES

1 CUP = 16 TABLESPOONS

1 CUP = 48 TEASPOONS

1 CUP = 1/2 PINT

1 CUP = 1/4 QUART

1 CUP = 1/16 GALLON

1 CUP = 240 ML

BAKING PAN CONVERSIONS

1 CUP ALL-PURPOSE FLOUR = 4.5 OZ

1 CUP ROLLED OATS = 3 OZ 1 LARGE EGG = 1.7 OZ

1 CUP BUTTER = 8 OZ 1 CUP MILK = 8 OZ

1 CUP HEAVY CREAM = 8.4 OZ

1 CUP GRANULATED SUGAR = 7.1 OZ

1 CUP PACKED BROWN SUGAR = 7.75 OZ

1 CUP VEGETABLE OIL = 7.7 OZ

1 CUP UNSIFTED POWDERED SUGAR = 4.4 OZ

BAKING PAN CONVERSIONS

9-INCH ROUND CAKE PAN = 12 CUPS

10-INCH TUBE PAN =16 CUPS

11-INCH BUNDT PAN = 12 CUPS

9-INCH SPRINGFORM PAN = 10 CUPS

9 X 5 INCH LOAF PAN = 8 CUPS

9-INCH SQUARE PAN = 8 CUPS

Appendix B : Recipes Index

P

Q

R

Made in the USA
Las Vegas, NV
05 January 2024

83972008R00059